The
# Glory
of the **Vision**

# The
# Glory
## of the Vision

Richard A. Schaefer

REVIEW AND HERALD® PUBLISHING ASSOCIATION

Since 1861 | www.reviewandherald.com

Review and Herald® titles may be purchased in bulk for educational, business, fund-raising, or sales promotional use. For information, e-mail SpecialMarkets@reviewandherald.com.

The Review and Herald® Publishing Association publishes biblically based materials for spiritual, physical, and mental growth and Christian discipleship.

The author assumes full responsibility for the accuracy of all facts and quotations as cited in this book. This book was condensed from the author's unabridged history of Loma Linda University which was edited by Dorothy Minchin-Comm.

This book was
Edited by Kalie Kelch
Copyedited by James Hoffer
Cover designed by Trent Truman
Interior designed by Tina M. Ivany
Cover photos by © istockphoto.com / salihguler / Greeek
Photos of Loma Linda University Medical Center: Supplied
Typeset: Bembo 11/14

PRINTED IN U.S.A.

14  13  12  11  10          5  4  3  2  1

Library of Congress Cataloging-in-Publication Data

Schaefer, Richard A.
   The glory of the vision : the incredible 100-year history of Loma Linda University School of Medicine / Richard A. Schaefer.
      p. ; cm.
1. Loma Linda University. School of Medicine—History. 2. Medical colleges—California—History. 3. Seventh-Day Adventist health facilities—California—History. I. Loma Linda University. School of Medicine. II. Title.
   [DNLM: 1. Protestantism—California. 2. Schools, Medical—history—California. 3. History, 20th Century—California. 4. History, 21st Century—California. 5. Religion and Medicine—California. W 19 S294g 2011]
   R746.C2S33 2011
   610.71'1794—dc22
                              2010021696

ISBN 978-0-8280-2479-2

Also by Richard A. Schaefer:

*On Becoming Shryock*

To order, call **1-800-765-6955**.
Visit us at **www.reviewandherald.com** for information on other
Review and Herald® products.

The Glory of the Vision, Book 2

is scheduled for release

Fall 2013.

# Letter to the Reader

During the beginning of our centennial celebration in 2009, I was asked by a newspaper reporter what was the most remarkable thing to happen to the Loma Linda University School of Medicine during its 100-year history. The answer was easy: Loma Linda University has remained tenaciously aligned with the mission and vision of its founder, Ellen G. White.

Ellen White instructed the school's leaders to do three things:

1. Teach its students not only how to manage the patients' physical and emotional needs but also how to understand and nurture the patients' *spiritual* needs. After all, most of us, when confronted with a life-threatening illness, will intrinsically turn to our spiritual side for guidance and comfort.

2. Prepare the students to become medical missionaries and take the health message and the promise of God's grace to the entire world. More than 1,000 of the medical school's graduates have served overseas—just how the school's founders envisioned.

3. Develop a medical school that will be "of the highest order." Our ability to educate excellent physicians has been an integral part of our reputation and verified by benchmark examinations.

*The Glory of the Vision* is about the miraculous feat of a few profoundly committed people of the Seventh-day Adventist Church who were directed by prayer and the Holy Spirit in the establishment and maturation of the Loma Linda University School of Medicine. In May 2011 the Loma Linda University School of Medicine will have graduated its 10,000th physician who was educated in a school whose mission has remained unchanged from its inception more than a century ago.

*The Glory of the Vision* is one of several books published by the School of Medicine commemorating its 100th anniversary, which will be celebrated from 2009 to 2014 (100 years from the matriculation of the first class to the first graduating class). Other books include the already-published and very popular *Morning Rounds*, a daily devotional book written by students, alumni, faculty, and friends of the Loma Linda University School of Medicine.

H. Roger Hadley, M.D.
Dean, Loma Linda University School of Medicine

# Contents

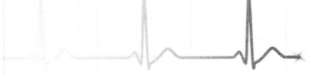

# Chapter 1

# A School of Medicine?

L oma Linda University is celebrating a milestone—100 years of service and education. As the largest school of medicine in California, with almost 700 currently enrolled medical students and approximately 10,000 physician graduates, Loma Linda University can be proud of its accomplishments. However, its humble beginnings tell a story of God's providence and leading. So how did it all start?

Loma Linda Sanitarium was scarcely operational when Ellen G. White, its cofounder, dispatched a letter to southern California. Now, for the first time, she mentioned her desire that Loma Linda should not only train nurses, but physicians as well. "Brother and Sister Burden, . . . In regard to the school, I would say, Make it all you possibly can in the education of nurses and physicians."[1]

Six months later, she repeated her instructions. Loma Linda was to be "not only a sanitarium, but also an educational center. . . . With the possession of this place comes the weighty responsibility of making the work of the institution educational in character. A school is to be established here for the training of gospel medical missionary evangelists."[2]

Identifying itself as a *Prospectus*, the institution's first bulletin declared the Loma Linda College of Evangelists affiliation with the Loma Linda Sanitarium. Then it described the kind of students Loma Linda wished to attract:

"Those who voluntarily and conscientiously commit themselves to the principles of trust-worthiness and faithfulness when no human eye is upon them, and who are willing to act in harmony with a common standard of right and expedience adopted by the school, even when it involves individual inconvenience. The effort will be, not to rule students, but to encourage and teach self-government. . . . Frivolous, sentimental, or undisciplined young people would not feel at home here, and would divert the energies of the school from its appointed work."[3]

The publication listed jewelry, showy ornaments, corsets, useless or hurtful reading, and bad habits under the heading "What to Leave at Home." It advised new students to send all "express matter" by Wells-Fargo, via Redlands Junction (formerly Bryn Mawr, now part of Loma Linda), California.[4]

### Academic Concerns

Ellen White recruited most of the professional faculty herself from around the United States. During the summer of 1906 a calendar was issued for the new school year. The following four courses were offered: Collegiate, Nurses, Gospel Workers, and a three-year Evangelistic-Medical course that included standard medical school class work plus Bible classes. Ellen White had counseled, "The healing of the sick and the ministry of the Word are to go hand in hand."[5] At 10:00 a.m., September 20, 1906, a portion of the faculty met for morning devotions and declared school in session; however, they did not have any students to teach. Fortunately, by October 4 the remainder of the faculty and approximately 35 students had arrived and instruction began.

Confused by the situation before him, John Burden, the business manager at Loma Linda, wrote to Ellen White on October 23 and asked for her counsel regarding the future curriculum of the college. Should the institution seek legal recognition as a school of medicine? Or should it seek legal recognition under a class of healer such as the homeopath, the chiropractor, or the osteopath? Or should it simply provide instruction for "medical evangelists," even though graduates would be unable legally to practice medicine?

Ellen White delayed her answer to his letter. Her personal desire was for Loma Linda to train physicians; however, at the time "The Battle Creek Syndrome," a label representing the church's response to the loss of the Battle Creek Sanitarium and its American Medical Missionary College (AMMC), still haunted the denomination. Perhaps the faith of the believers needed to be strengthened even more. As they observed God's providential guidance in the months ahead, they would unite and sacrifice to establish a well-equipped, properly staffed school of medicine. A year later, when Burden again asked whether the school was "simply to qualify nurses" or whether it should "embrace also the qualification for physicians," she replied, "Physicians are to receive their education here."[6]

## Financial Worries

In 1907 a nationwide depression further impacted the financial stability of the Loma Linda Sanitarium. Because the institution could not pay even modest wages and salaries, it compensated the personnel (called "helpers") and medical staff with aluminum tokens. Only the store, the dairy, and the employees' dining room accepted these tokens. During this time, teams of volunteer physicians, nurses, and students conducted "schools of health" in private homes. There they taught basic rules of healthful living, hygiene, and nutrition to groups of up to 20 people. With the blessings of local public school authorities, these teams delivered health lectures in nearby San Bernardino elementary schools and high schools. They also distributed a special health-and-temperance issue of the denomination's magazine, *The Youths' Instructor*.

In February 1908, 17 months after the College of Evangelists opened, a local committee met in Loma Linda to study relationships among the educational institutions in southern California. Obviously, some young people should be educated as fully accredited physicians. The committee, however, estimated that laboratories and other needed facilities for a medical school would cost $40,000 to $50,000—more than the original cost of the sanitarium. When asked whether the needed facilities should be provided, Ellen White cautioned against premature action: "The plans you suggest seem to be essential, but you need to assure yourselves that they can be safely carried. . . . If you had the talent and means to carry such responsibilities, we should be glad to see your plans carry."[7]

## Preparing the Way

Ellen White cautioned that establishing a large medical school would depend on the church members' united effort. A month later she wrote, "We should not at this time seek to compete with worldly medical schools . . . [because]

our chances of success would be small. We are not now prepared to carry out successfully the work of establishing large medical institutions of learning."[8]

In 1909 the Loma Linda College of Evangelists continued its three-year evangelistic-medical course. The faculty could only encourage those who wanted to become physicians to hope that their education would be accepted as equivalent to the first two years at public schools of medicine or that it would count toward graduation at Loma Linda, should it eventually become an accredited school of medicine.

## A Significant Conversation

In September of that year Burden interviewed Ellen White and shared with her the concerns of the faculty and students. She replied that the church should "have a school of [its] own" to educate physicians and that it would not be a violation of principle to obtain a charter. Following is an excerpt from their conversation:

**Burden**: "The governments of earth provide that if we conduct a medical school, we must take a charter from the government. That in itself has nothing to do with how the school is conducted. It is required, however, that certain studies shall be taught. There are ten required subjects. Physiology is one of these. It is required that those who labor as physicians shall be proficient in these subjects. In starting our sanitariums for the care of the sick, we must secure a charter from the government. . . . Would the securing of a charter for a medical school, where our students might obtain a medical education, militate against our depending upon God?"

**White**: "No; I do not see that it would, if a charter were secured on the right terms. Only be sure that you do not exalt men above God. If you can gain force and influence that will make your work more effective, without tying yourself to worldly men, that would be right. . . ."

**Burden**: "The only thing that we have asked for in this matter is to take advantage of the government provision that would give standing room to our students when they are qualified."

**White**: "I do not see anything wrong in that. . . . You may unite with them in certain points that will not have a misleading influence, but let no sacrifice be made to endanger our principles. We shall always have to stand distinct.

God desires us to be separate, and yet it is our privilege to avail ourselves of certain rights. . . ."

**Burden**: "It seems clear to me that any standing we can lawfully have without compromising is not out of harmony with God's plan."

**White**: "No; it is not."[9]

Five weeks later, she enlarged the concept in a letter to Burden: "Wise laws have been framed in order to safeguard our people against the imposition of unqualified physicians. These laws we should respect, for we are ourselves by them protected from presumptuous pretenders. Should we manifest opposition to these requirements, it would tend to restrict the influence of our medical missionaries."[10]

## Structuring the New College

Despite seemingly immovable obstacles, the administration of the school decided to follow the counsel of Ellen White and establish a school of medicine for Seventh-day Adventists. Church leaders then changed the school's name from the College of Evangelists to the College of Medical Evangelists (CME), which was incorporated under the laws of the state of California on Thursday, December 9, 1909.[11] The state of California granted the charter on December 13.[12] The new corporation was to exist "for fifty years and for such further time as shall be allowed by law."[13]

## Providential Additions to the Faculty: The Sixth Physician

The College of Medical Evangelists began with just five physicians. Within three weeks of the December 9, 1909, charter, a sixth physician joined the faculty: Dr. Alfred Q. Shryock.[14] All, however, were general practitioners—not a promising start for a school of medicine. This inauspicious beginning is a continuing witness to the providential heritage of Loma Linda.

When Alfred Shryock graduated from the American Medical Missionary College (AMMC) in Battle Creek, Michigan (1899), he was president of his senior class. His wife, Stella, completed nurses' training at the Battle Creek Sanitarium before the couple married in 1899. Both were second generation Adventists. Alfred Shryock, now a practicing physician, believed that it was more important to help people rather than to gain wealth. In 1900, after teaching for one year at AMMC, he accepted an invitation from the Washington Conference of Seventh-day Adventists to direct a church-owned hydrotherapy treatment unit in Seattle.

Alfred Shryock moved the hydrotherapy unit to a better location, appointed Stella as supervisor and receptionist, and eventually employed several other nurses and a "lady physician." The unit flourished as it treated patients suffering from upper respiratory infections. Alfred Shryock also commuted by boat every two weeks to supervise a similar unit operated by a nurse in Bellingham, Washington. By 1908 Alfred Shryock had become somewhat prosperous. He had established a substantial family medicine practice, associated it with the hydrotherapy unit, and built a new home on Queen Anne Hill, a residential suburb of Seattle.

The Shryock's winter vacation took them and their 2-year-old son, Harold, to southern California. They wanted to visit some of the Seventh-day Adventist sanitariums being developed there. Because of its controversial beginning, church members generally considered the Loma Linda Sanitarium to be of special interest, perhaps even somewhat sensational.

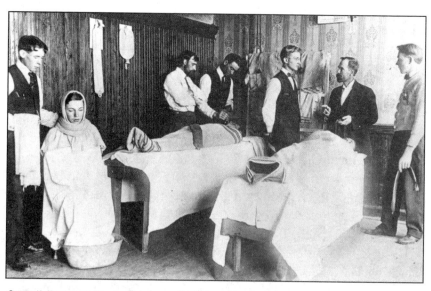

George K. Abbott, M.D., teaches techniques of hydrotherapy in October 1909. At 26, Abbott was the youngest president of CME. He spent 32 years in service to SDA health institutions, during which time he actively promoted a vigorous health program.

Most of the institution's five physicians had been Alfred Shryock's schoolmates at AMMC. They expressed their strong faith that the new institution was under a divine mandate. Then came the big news. They were about to organize a school of medicine. They had based their plans on Ellen White's recent statement that "physicians are to receive their education here [at Loma Linda]."[15]

Dr. George K. Abbott, president of the sanitarium and college, remembered that Alfred Shryock had had some experience teaching at AMMC, and he urged him to "come and join us."[16] Specifically, he wanted Alfred Shryock to teach courses in histology and human embryology. (Alfred Shryock had worked for Dr. A. B. Olson at AMMC as a student laboratory assistant for a course in histology.)

On their way back to Seattle, Alfred Shryock rejected the idea of successfully starting a school of medicine in Loma Linda as an unrealistic hope. The very idea of a medical school was incredibly ambitious, considering that the sanitarium was still struggling for its very existence. "I really don't care to be affiliated," he told Stella, "with a one-horse medical school."

Nevertheless, the motivated and persistent physicians at Loma Linda continued their appeals by mail. "We believe the plan to develop a school here for the training of gospel medical missionary evangelists is divinely ordained," they insisted. Although the sincerity of the Loma Linda physicians impressed the Shryocks, it did not persuade them to leave Seattle.

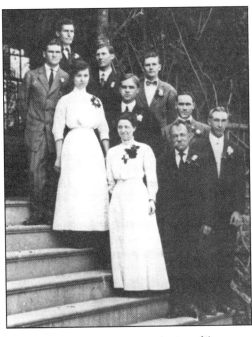

CME's first student physicians pose on the steps of the Assembly Hall with Bible teacher Roderick S. Owen.

Burden offered Alfred Shryock a salary of $20 per week. When Alfred Shryock replied that he would be unable to meet his expenses on $20 per week, Burden replied that after due consideration he would offer him $21 a week.

Finally, being conscientious, the Shryocks thought, "maybe the Lord's hand *is* in this." So they prayed for a sign. If God wanted them to move to Loma Linda, He would need to send a buyer for their new home. That would be an impressive and useful sign. Alfred Shryock listed the property with a realtor on his way to work one morning. Miraculously, the new home sold before noon, and by sundown that same day, it was in escrow. Providence had made it perfectly clear what direction the family's future would take. At a cost of $148.10, Alfred Shryock moved his small family to southern California and became Loma Linda's sixth physician.

State law established CME's admission requirements, and the Association of American Medical Colleges set its academic standards. (Students not possessing high school or academic diplomas accompanied by a certified statement of the requirements had to be evaluated by an examiner appointed by the State Board of Medical Examiners.) Abbott provided prospective students with all of the details and requirements.[17]

Shortly after CME's incorporation, the Pacific Union Conference met on January 25, 1910, at Mountain View, California, for its fifth biennial session. They decided that in order to support such an ambitious enterprise, church officials must be satisfied that they correctly understood Ellen White's counsel. The next day they gave Ellen White a letter asking a very pertinent question:

"Are we to understand, from what you have written concerning the establishment of a medical school at Loma Linda, that, according to the light you have received from the Lord, we are to establish a thoroughly equipped medical school, the graduates from which will be able to take state board examinations and become registered, qualified physicians?"[18]

## A College of the Highest Order

Ellen White's equally specific reply went out the next day:

"The light given me is [that] we must provide that which is essential to qualify our youth who desire to be physicians, so that they may intelligently fit themselves to be able to stand the examinations required to prove their efficiency as physicians. They should be taught to treat understandingly the cases of those who are diseased, so that the door will be closed for any sensible physician to imagine that we are not giving in our school the instruction necessary for properly qualifying young men and young women to do the work of a physician. . . . The medical school at Loma Linda is to be of the highest order.

"And for the special preparation of those of our youth who have clear convictions of their duty to obtain a medical education that will enable them to pass the examinations required by law of all those who practice as regularly qualified physicians, we are to supply whatever may be required, so that these youth need not be compelled to go to medical schools conducted by men not of our faith.

"[Moreover], whatever subjects are required[19] as essential in the [medical] schools conducted by those not of our faith, we are to supply [to the church's youth]. . . . [They must] obtain a medical education that will enable them to pass the examinations required by law of all those who practice as regularly qualified physicians."[20]

Establishing such a school, of course, would require the broad-based financial support of the entire denomination. Pastor I. H. Evans, a vice president of the General Conference, spoke enthusiastically of advancing by faith.

"We have before us . . . a plain, straightforward statement from Sister White, in regard to the establishment of a medical school. There is no guesswork about it; there is no equivocation; there is no false construction that need be put upon these words. The question is, Will we follow the counsel given?

"I can conjure up many reasons why at this time we are ill-prepared to establish and operate a medical school. It is not hard for any man to say that we have not the money at hand. Any man need not be very wise to say, 'We do not know where we shall get medical men trained and qualified to take up this work.' But the question is, Will we establish this medical school, when the Lord has indicated so plainly our duty? I believe, brethren, if we step forward in the fear of God, and make an effort to establish this school, the Lord will help us and make the way clear."[21]

At the conclusion of this discussion, the question was called, and the vote of the delegates upon the recommendation under discussion was *unanimous.* At the request of the delegates, the question was then submitted to the whole house for their action, and a similar vote was cast.[22]

During this meeting, the General Conference of Seventh-day Adventists and the Pacific Union Conference assumed ownership of the College of Medical Evangelists.[23] Church members responded with a heartfelt enthusiasm that ensured united action on behalf of the new medical college. Still, "the rivers of difficulties were full and overflowing their banks," as Dr. Percy T. Magan, an early administrator at Loma Linda, would later describe the situation. Indeed, none believed they had sufficient financial resources or talents to undertake the enterprise. Still, many believed God had shown them that the time was right. They responded to His call with the few resources they had, believing He would bless and multiply. They believed He had called the church to take this leap of faith.

## How Near Is Our End to Our Beginning?

Incorporated on December 9, 1909, as part of the College of Medical Evangelists, the infant medical school could not have been born into a colder legal climate. In 1910 the Abraham Flexner Report, financed by the Carnegie Foundation for the Advancement of Teaching, continued what the AMA's Council on Medical Education had started in 1906. It promoted the closing of inadequate medical schools in the United States. Strict new accreditation procedures graded each surviving school and closed those that did not measure up. By 1932 authorities had closed a sobering 84 schools of medicine in the United States.[24]

Years later, Dr. Edward Sutherland, who had attended medical school at the University of Tennessee and Vanderbilt University, spoke of the upheaval:

"They intended to see that only one medical college should exist in [each] state unless a university and a private medical school, then they would let two. But they would not allow more than two medical schools in the same state. They intended to bring the standard up. And I want to say that they did so because there was a great deal of cheap, mercenary business in medical schools. They'd even sell diplomas. Things were in horrible shape, and so they did a fine piece of cleansing."[25]

Accreditation authorities told CME administrators that it would be impossible for a new, poorly equipped, church-related school of medicine to measure up to these strict standards. In his book, *For God and C.M.E.*, Merlin L. Neff provides a valuable historical perspective:

"In 1910 few Seventh-day Adventists comprehended what was happening in medical education in the United States. They saw little need to pour money into the construction of classrooms, laboratories, and hospitals. Church leaders knew of many physicians who, by taking short courses, had received the M.D. degree. Furthermore, it had been possible for a young man to be trained in medicine by any physician who would act as his preceptor. Some argued that the young people should take short courses in medical evangelism, as they did in ministerial training, to prepare them for foreign-mission service.

**AMA Requirements for a Legitimate Medical College (by Nathan Colwell)**

- A large campus
- Adequate library
- Laboratories (pharmacology and pathology)
- Classrooms
- A 100-bed hospital[28]
- Many specialists in each branch of medicine
- Strong financial backing

"[Now] high standards of training were suddenly demanded, and adequate laboratories and hospitals were declared essential for CME. Leaders in the North American Division [of the denomination] balked [however] at appropriating the funds called for to carry on a medical college."[26]

On April 27, 1910, Ellen White wrote Burden a long letter calling for independence from worldly men and organizations. Her objections focused on ungodly or worldly teachers who had peculiar prejudices. But she promoted medical missionaries who would become efficient by being diligent in study and faithful in service.

"We should have in various places, men of extraordinary ability, who have obtained their diplomas in medical schools of the best reputation who can stand before the world as fully qualified and legally recognized physicians. Let God-fearing men be wisely chosen to go through the training essential in order to obtain such qualifications."[27]

In the spring of 1910 Arthur G. Daniells, president of the General Conference, traveled to Loma Linda for a reincorporation meeting to join the Loma Linda Sanitarium and the College of Medical Evangelists. Concerned that Burden would commit the church to an overwhelming financial obligation, Daniells took "back-up" with him—Professor Homer

Salisbury, secretary of education for the General Conference. The two men stopped in Chicago to visit Dr. Nathan P. Colwell, secretary of the American Medical Association Council on Medical Education. Colwell had been authorized to examine and rate medical schools and to enforce AMA requirements.

Hoping not to prejudice Colwell against Loma Linda, they identified themselves by name only. Deliberately they said nothing about Loma Linda or their church. They would do nothing to jeopardize the possibility of the denomination's starting an AMA-accredited medical school. They simply asked what facilities would be needed to establish an acceptable medical college.

Daniells and Salisbury thanked Colwell and started to leave. Jumping to his feet, Colwell pointed at Daniells, "And you tell those people at Loma Linda these facts!"

"What makes you think we are from Loma Linda?" Daniells inquired.

"Because," Colwell answered, "Nobody in the world is so foolish as to think you can build and maintain a medical college without money, except you Adventists!"

"Well, Dr. Colwell, suppose we put it on anyway?" asked Daniells.

"You put it on," Colwell snapped, "and we will put it off. We are *not* going to have any more of these 'one-horse' medical schools in this country!"[29]

What to do? Colwell's "laundry list" looked very challenging.

## Fine-tuning the Administration

Well, the Adventists decided to "put it on anyway" with a new corporation consolidating the sanitarium and the college and their respective boards of trustees. How could they take such a bold step—virtually an act of defiance?

The instruction from Ellen White had been so definite that the committee on plans and recommendations voted that the new school be established on a broader and firmer basis. They recommended that the General Conference and the union conferences all give support to the project.[30] The General Conference set the proposal before its Spring Council in April 1910.

The next order of business was to choose CME's president. On May 11, 1910, the board of trustees elected Dr. Wells A. Ruble, medical secretary of the General Conference, as president of the medical college.[31]

## Applying the "Testimonies" to CME

Ellen White's latest statements had been so detailed that Board Chair George A. Irwin published a 20-page leaflet outlining the group's thinking: "The latest communications [from Ellen G. White] in regard to this enterprise were so clear and explicit that all doubt as to their intent was removed from the minds of the members of the council; and hence, from the very beginning, the meeting was characterized by a spirit of earnestness and determination on the part of all to move out at once upon the instruction received. The launching of such an enterprise being a new

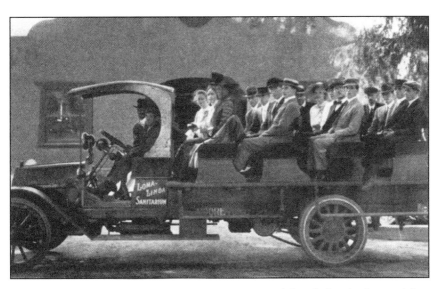

Faculty and students ride in the "air conditioned" Moore truck to an evangelistic-medical meeting. Accommodating 21 passengers, the truck transported students to and from the San Bernardino County Hospital.

thing in our experience, we had to feel our way along step by step; and while each proposed move was discussed freely, an excellent spirit prevailed, and when an action was passed it was by the unanimous vote of all the delegation."[32]

Having two corporations doing the work the Testimonies said should be done by *one* motivated the council to recommend consolidation. Therefore, on May 11, 1910, the CME board of trustees merged the two corporations into one: "[We believe] that greater efficiency and simplicity in the administration of its educational interests will result therefrom by such consolidation of the two organizations under our management." Identified as "The Corporation of the College of Medical Evangelists," the new board consisted of 21 members, each serving three-year terms of office.[33] Seven members constituted a quorum for the transaction of business, and the corporation was to "exist for fifty years from and after the date of consolidation."

The committee on plans and recommendations also found other ways to generate income. They proposed new fees for the medical school: $100 per year for tuition (up from $75), $5 per year for matriculation, $1 per year for the use of the library, and $10 for graduation. Finally, they also suggested that the medical school openly solicit contributions for its operating costs. [34]

### Curriculum

Medical school applicants had to present a "Medical Students' Certificate," preferably from the Michigan State Board, stating that they had completed the required courses for admission to the institution. In lieu of this they could obtain a certificate from another state board. Failure to obtain this document meant that students had to have their credentials verified by the examiner of entrance credentials to medical schools for southern California.

In addition to the studies prescribed by the American Medical Association

| Required Courses for Admission to CME | CME's First Curriculum | |
|---|---|---|
| Mathematics and Advanced Mathematics | Bible | |
| Latin | Pastoral Training | |
| Physics | Anatomy | Physiology |
| History | Chemistry | Histology |
| Languages | Hydrotherapy | Mechanic Therapy |
| English and Literature | Embryology | Bandaging |
| Natural Sciences | Pharmacology | Mat[eria] Med[ica] |
| Physical Sciences | Food/Dietetics | Physical Diagnosis |
| Physiology | Gynecology | Obstetrics |
| Hygiene | The Practice of Medicine[37] | |
| Drawing | | |

and the Association of American Medical Colleges, CME emphasized hydrotherapy and allied subjects as well as Bible study, thus lengthening the medical course work to *five* years.[35] Ellen White's counsels and the unique but successful operation of Seventh-day Adventist sanitariums around the world influenced CME's curriculum, which was evident in the institution's bulletin: "The Medical Course extends over five years of thirty-six weeks each. While the medical course as ordinarily given in medical schools lasts only four years, it is manifestly impossible to crowd into this time all that should be given in medical and scientific lines together with Bible, evangelistic training, hydrotherapy, and dietetics and also provide for a practical experience in the diagnosis and treatment of disease under competent instruction as called for by the curriculum."[36]

Practical experience was obtained through interaction in treatment rooms, the sanitarium laboratory, the pharmacy, and the operating room. Students gained experience by caring for the sick, diagnosing illnesses, and prescribing treatments. Because electric lights had not yet been perfected, the first operating room on the third floor of the sanitarium had inadequate lighting. Although gas lights were the brightest, fear of explosion from the type of anesthetics used at that time precluded their use. Therefore, surgeons scheduled their operations during the brightest time of the day and illuminated their surgeries by sunlight from nearby windows.[38]

The next year CME added to its curriculum pathology, autopsies, surgery, pediatrics, diseases of the eye, ear, nose, and throat, genito-urinary diseases, mental, nervous diseases, dermatology, syphilis, electrotherapy, hygiene, and medical jurisprudence. To its practical experience it added anesthesia and operating assistance, autopsies and clinical microscopy, electro and radiotherapy, general evangelistic, field work, gospel talks and Bible reading, and health and temperance talks.[39]

Because administrators obviously envisioned CME as a resource for the entire denomination, they emphasized its missionary focus. Students quickly noticed CME's unique curriculum and outlook. For example, Fred Herzer, a second-year medical student who had transferred from another school of medicine, compared his experience at both institutions. His statement confirmed the denomination's rationale for starting CME. He began by expressing his disappointing experience at the first school.

## What Makes CME Unique?

I [Fred Herzer] entered with the intent to obtain a knowledge that would place me in a position to be of more benefit to my fellow men. I expected to obtain a fuller knowledge of the manifestation of the power of God in the human body.

Before the end of the first year as a medical student, I was sadly disappointed, and must say disgusted, with the whole thing. The charm of the work had lessened materially. To some extent, at least, I can directly account for the unexpected change. From the association with classmates, instructors and various experiences, especially in the dissecting room, my reverence for humanity was materially lowered, and the feeling of sacredness for death lessened.

From numerous lectures by "brainy men" on the theories of evolution and mechanism, I must admit that my former belief in the "seven-day-creation" plan was decidedly shaken. They argued cunningly and forcibly that all natural phenomena could be accounted for by physical and mechanical laws—that the animate by slow gradation had developed from the inanimate. When so-called church members, Christians, if you please, take such a position, it is difficult under a long course of study not to be harmed by it to some extent at least. The Bible had no place whatsoever, and its principles were denied in more ways than one.

What a contrast in the spirit and atmosphere of the medical students at this place. All are working eagerly to obtain that medical evangelical education which will fit them for the work of carrying the last gospel to the world, all with a high sense of morality, all holding the life of mankind in high reverence, and all feeling a reverence for death. They are not a class of students looking at the profession from a financial standpoint.

We feel and know that our instructors are intensely interested in our welfare; they are not men and women teaching the theories of physiologic principles and wholly disregarding them in their own lives. Ours is the privilege of attending this new, "only-one-of-the-kind," best medical college on earth, giving the Bible the first place, and advancing according to direct Testimony.[40]

A major problem had not yet been addressed. What about the 100-bed clinical hospital? True, all of these other activities supported the continuing ministry of CME, but, nonetheless, the most pressing need was to provide facilities for students to obtain more clinical education. The sanitarium served ambulatory/rehabilitation patients. A hospital would provide facilities to treat bed-ridden patients—those recovering from surgery, those who had serious injuries, or those who suffered from acute illnesses and diseases. In the first move to establish a hospital, on April 18, 1911, the board voted to move surgery from the sanitarium to the west rooms on the first floor of the large cottage on the hill. The move was scheduled for completion by November 1, 1911.[41]

## The AMA and Dr. Colwell—Again

In the late fall of 1911 Colwell visited CME to make a preliminary assessment of its standing with the American Medical Association. He seemed pleased with CME's progress in teaching basic sciences. He could not yet make a report, however, because the school was conducting classes in but three of its five-year curriculum.[42]

Colwell had apparently not changed his mind since his earlier conversation with Daniells and Salisbury the previous year. "Why are you starting a new school when there are already 150 medical schools in the United States? Don't you know we are endeavoring to reduce the number of such colleges by cutting out the small schools that are not well prepared to give medical training?" By way of reply, Ruble presented him with the five unique objectives of the new school.

After examining the school and conferring with its faculty, Colwell met with Burden. Funding seemed to be his greatest concern. "What is the financial backing of this school?"

**Objectives for the College of Medical Evangelists (1911)**

1. To prepare medical missionaries to go into foreign lands to preach the gospel.

2. To provide a school where we can educate our own Seventh-day Adventist people for our own work.

3. To give to young people a training in the special lines of treatment which we pursue in our denominational institutions that are scattered around the world.

4. To throw around our students an influence tending to keep them true to their determination to prepare themselves for medical missionary work.

5. To provide a first-class medical college where our young people may get a medical education without being obliged to violate their consciences by engaging in work on the seventh day of the week.

Burden replied that the church's 110,000 members made up any deficits in its mission and educational programs. He further explained how church members had successfully supported various financial projects that had seemed, to all human appearances, doomed to failure. Burden then described the unique *physical, mental,* and *spiritual* emphasis of the church's international missionary program and said, "Will you tell me, doctor, to what school can we send our young people to equip them for this world mission work with this threefold preparation?"

Colwell replied, "There is no such school in existence."

Burden then asked, "Do you propose to destroy this little medical school ... that is in no way competing with your endowed medical colleges, but is our only means for supplying our missionary program?"

At first, Colwell answered indirectly. "Mr. Burden, when I took my medical course it was to become a medical missionary. . . . The medical got me, and the mission lost out."[43] In the end, he clearly understood CME's needs. From that day onward Colwell befriended CME. He understood its purposes and was in full sympathy with its objectives.[44]

[1]Ellen G. White, letter 325, December 10, 1905.

[2]Ellen G. White, "Dedication of the Loma Linda Sanitarium," *Review and Herald,* June 21, 1906, p. 8.

[3]Loma Linda College of Evangelists, Prospectus, 1906-1907, Loma Linda, California, p. 21.

[4]*Ibid.*, pp. 23, 24.

[5]Ellen G. White, "Special Work at Loma Linda," *Testimonies and Experiences Connected With the Loma Linda Sanitarium and College of Medical Evangelists,* Loma Linda, California, p. 23.

[6]Ellen G. White, October 30, 1907, MS 151, 1907 (*Medical Ministry,* p. 76).

[7]Ellen G. White, letter 82, 1908.

[8]Ellen G. White, letter 90, 1908.

[9]"The Relation of Loma Linda College to Worldly Medical Institutions," Ellen G. White interview by John A. Burden, September 23, 1909, MS 72, 1909, Paulson Collection, pp. 269-274; "J. A. Burden Seeks Counsel Regarding Legal Recognition and a Charter," September 20, 1909.

[10]Ellen G. White, letter (140) to John A. Burden, November 5, 1909.

[11]The incorporation meeting convened at 2:00 p.m. at the Southern California Conference office, 424 Broadway Street, in Los Angeles, California. First Meeting of Incorporation of College of Medical Evangelists, minutes, December 9, 1909, p. 1.

[12]"History," *Loma Linda University Magazine,* spring 1965, p. 38.

[13]Second Meeting of Incorporation of College of Medical Evangelists, *Articles of Incorporation of the College of Medical Evangelists,* pp. 1-5.

[14]The charter of December 9, 1909, legalized the college.

[15]Ellen G. White, October 30, 1907, manuscript 151, 1907. (*Medical Ministry,* p. 76).

[16]George Abbott was a 1903 graduate of AMMC. He served as medical superintendent of the Loma Linda Sanitarium and also president of the College of Medical Evangelists.

[17]"College of Medical Evangelists," *The Medical Evangelist*, fourth quarter, 1909, p. 36.

[18]I. H. Evans, E. E. Andross, H. W. Cottrell, letter, "A Letter of Inquiry," *Pacific Union Recorder*, February 3, 1910, pp. 2, 3; "A Medical School at Loma Linda," *Review and Herald*, May 19, 1910, pp. 17, 18; D. E. Robinson, "A Bold Venture in Faith," *The Story of Our Health Message*, pp. 383-385; *Loma Linda Messages* (Payson, Arizona: Leaves of Autumn, 1973), pp. 484, 485.

[19]In these words is found the justification for accrediting Seventh-day Adventist educational institutions, a point made in *Counsels to Parents and Teachers*: "Our larger union conference training schools should be placed in the most favorable position for qualifying our youth to meet the entrance requirements specified by state laws regarding medical students." Ellen G. White, *Counsels to Parents and Teachers*, p. 479.

[20]Ellen G. White, "Testimonies and Experiences Connected With The Loma Linda Sanitarium and the College of Medical Evangelists," *Medical Evangelistic Library*, No. 1, pp. 5, 15.

[21]I. H. Evans, "Advancing by Faith," *Pacific Union Recorder*, February 3, 1910, p. 8.

[22]The Ellen G. White Publications, General Conference, Washington, D.C., "Medical Practice and the Educational Program at Loma Linda, A Compilation of Ellen G. White Counsels Supplemented With Illuminating Statements of Denominational Leader and Significant Committee and Constituency Actions," March 1972, p. 92.

[23]"The Purchase of Land at Loma Linda," *Special Testimonies*, Series B, No. 17, p. 3.

[24]S. Jonas, *Medical Mystery: The Training of Doctors in the United States* (New York: W. W. Norton and Company, 1978), p. 223; Association of American Medical Colleges, "Final Report of the Commission on Medical Education," 1932, appendix tables 60 and 104; U. S. Department of Commerce, "Statistical Abstract of the United States," 1974, table 2; Louis L. Smith, M.D., "Research in the Clinical Departments," *Diamond Memories*, p. 179.

[25]Edward Sutherland, M.D. Loma Linda Volunteer Fire Chief Francis Dinsmore documented this report on a wire recording at a Camp Cedar Falls retreat in 1949; Centennial Anniversary of CME/LLU—2005, Department of Archives and Special Collections, Document File 3229.06.

[26]Merlin L. Neff, "A Medical School in the West," *For God and C.M.E.* (Mountain View, California: Pacific Press Publishing Association, 1964), p. 164.

[27]Ellen G. White, letter (61) to John Burden, April 27, 1910.

[28]The 100-bed hospital needed to be located in a poverty-stricken section of some city. It would provide clinical experience for the students.

[29]Owen S. Parrett, M.D., "Daniells and Salisbury Visit Colwell," *Stories of the Early College of Medical Evangelists*, pp. 110, 111.

[30]The union conferences included: the Lake, Northern, Central, Southwestern, and North Pacific. The Southern California Conference was asked to join the Pacific Union Conference in financially supporting the institution.

[31] CME board of trustees, minutes, May 11, 1910, p. 22.

[32] G. A. Irwin, "A Brief History and Some Facts Relative to the College of Medical Evangelists," pp. 8, 9, White Document File 392.

[33] The term of office for each board member began and ended August 24 every year. The Loma Linda Sanitarium had been incorporated on August 24, 1905. CME board of trustees, minutes, May 11, 1910, pp. 48-52.

[34]*Ibid.*, May 9, 1910, pp. 1, 2.

[35]*The Medical Evangelist*, vol. 3, No. 2, February 1911, p. 26.

[36]*The College of Medical Evangelists Bulletin*, 1911-1912, pp. 16, 17.

[37] *The Medical Evangelist*, vol. 1, No. 5, fourth quarter, 1909, p. 35.

[38] Raymond E. Ryckman, Ph.D., "Early Years at Loma Linda," *Edmund C. Jaeger, Son of the Living Desert, 1887-1983*, p. 29.

[39] "The Second Annual Announcement of the College of Medical Evangelists," 1910-1911, p. 15.

[40] Fred Herzer, *The Medical Evangelist*, February 1911, pp. 17, 18.

[41] CME board of trustees, minutes, April 18, 1911, p. 139.

[42] *The Medical Evangelist*, October-November 1911, p. 135.

[43] John Burden, letter to E. H. Risley, M.D., June 3, 1929.

[44] *The Medical Evangelist*, January 1912, pp. 17, 18.

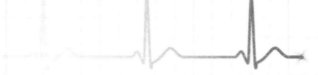

# Chapter 2:

# A Year of Impossibilities, 1912

In order to succeed, CME would need advanced ratings from the Council on Medical Education. That, however, was but half the story. It also had to have the tireless support of the entire Seventh-day Adventist denomination. Records from 1912 indicate a mix of staggering problems, strong faith, and a raw instinct for survival. The leadership believed, however, that CME would be of great significance to the Adventist Church.

### The General Conference President Speaks

In January 1913 the AMA's Council on Medical Education surveyed the College of Medical Evangelists. It had not yet, however, graded the school.[1] While this might be interpreted as a step forward, Irwin, the General Conference president, had already set the sobering facts before the constituency meeting the previous year.

His report illustrates the dynamics within the denomination that influenced the fledgling institution and envisioned its future:

"The launching of this enterprise was one of the most important moves made by this denomination . . . the beginning of a work that will have a world-wide influence for good, if the object and principles of the promoters are kept ever in view and rigorously maintained. . . . While this institution is located within the bounds of the Southern California Conference and the Pacific Union Conference it is not in any sense a local enterprise. It is the only school of its kind in the whole denomination, and hence of general interest to all parts of the great field."

## The Campaign for a Hospital Begins

Ruble added that the college required the "same standards as the AMA." Ideally this would be the case, but a major difficulty stood in the way. The Loma Linda Sanitarium, albeit successful, was *not* a hospital. Although it had almost 100 patients, for a variety of reasons it did not fulfill the school's needs.

First, the patronage fluctuated with the seasons. Second, the spectrum of conditions did not include many surgical cases, and almost no obstetrical cases. Last, both staff and patients were convinced that those who paid full rates for their care should not be questioned and probed by student physicians. All were persuaded that CME needed a "charity" hospital to provide "hands-on" education for the medical students.

Amidst the difficulties and challenges of establishing a hospital, one of many positive outcomes was the fact that Seventh-day Adventist church members could receive the best medical attention at a moderate cost at the new hospital proposed for CME.[2] At that time scores of church members sought help at other hospitals because they could not afford to pay sanitarium rates.

As usual, Ellen White remained central to all CME plans. The next day she spoke for 30 minutes, emphasizing the fact that members of the constituency were working for time and eternity. The spirit of cooperation that had characterized the councils pleased her, and she declared that unity would be essential in accomplishing the great work before the group. Indeed, harmony would encourage the blessing of God. She concluded with a statement that had both practical and prophetic implications. She urged the importance of holding all the land they possessed. "We shall need it all. We may not see this now, but we shall see it in the future."[3]

## Struggling With the Great Hurdle

In order to provide clinical experience to student physicians, CME desperately needed to build its own hospital as soon as possible. On May 27, 1912, "the committee on hospital" reported:

"On account of the necessity for clinical opportunity for the college next year, it was moved by Abbott, seconded by Salisbury, to construct a hospital for clinical purposes, consisting in general of a clinical part 46 feet by 72 feet, and two wings to be used as wards; the north wing to be built as soon as funds can be raised for the purpose. The entire hospital shall be one story, and the clinical portion at least constructed of concrete. Carried! The board also voted that some of the physicians be relieved for the summer so that they could go on the road and solicit funds for CME."[4]

The board recommended another option for providing the vital clinical experience.

They recommended on May 31, 1912, that physicians in the sanitarium make use of students in their fourth and fifth years of study as office assistants, to provide "as thorough a practical experience as is consistent with the highest ideals of medical ethics." They voted that any physician who had an important case could conduct a clinic, as arranged with management, and to confine obstetrics and gynecology clinical work to fourth- and fifth-year students. They also voted to arrange for fourth- and fifth-year students to become interns in sister sanitariums for two or more weeks per year and to spend as much time as possible during vacations. Furthermore, they authorized management to arrange for students to receive clinical experience locally at the San Bernardino County Hospital (San Bernardino) and at Patton State Hospital (Highland).[5]

Then, of course, the tuition income came up for discussion again. The cost had risen from $100 to $150. Even with tight finances, however, Burden felt that the proposed increase for medical students was excessive. On June 17, 1912, he reported that the tuition in other medical schools averaged $122. He recommended that CME tuition remain at $100 with the addition of a $10 laboratory fee. His motion carried.[6]

The board inspected CME's facilities, including its laboratories, library, courses of study, and clinical facilities. They noted its recognition by other medical schools and the Association of American Medical Colleges. They acknowledged its efficient faculty and the substantial plans for the future. Then they voted to recommend to Seventh-day Adventist young people who anticipated becoming physicians that they attend CME rather than any other institution. "We believe [that] by so doing that they will be far more efficiently prepared for work in this Great Advent Movement."[7]

## A Depressing Turn of Events

In the midst of this momentum, December 1912 found the college scrambling. The funds had failed to materialize. With its back up against the wall CME suspended all improvements, except a few very urgent ones. Fiscal responsibility prevailed. The board did not want to proceed with construction until the funds were in hand. With considerable anxiety the board explained their action: "We recognize that this is a very hazardous thing to do for the interest of our College, being it is time now when the Hospital should be at the present time in use for the good of the College. This step is liable to place our College in a class that will work great harm to our school, but the Board felt that until further means is in hand we cannot go further."[8]

In January 1913 the constituency held a special meeting to take advantage of the fact that the General Conference Committee was meeting in Mountain View (January 19 to 25). It invited members of the Canadian conferences to participate in the deliberations. Local members of the board urged this meeting in order to benefit from the advice and counsel of the General Conference Committee, who composed a large part of CME's constituency. Because of insufficient notice to make the meeting legal, the group passed on many important matters that could be ratified by the regular legal meeting that would be held the fourth Wednesday in March.[9]

Again, the group confronted its crisis—how to provide facilities for CME to qualify for a good rating from the AMA. The ownership and control of a properly equipped and managed clinical hospital along with an outpatient dispensary would determine CME's future success. It could rise or fall on this one point. Irwin reminded them of Ellen White's dedicated involvement with CME. She had "visited Loma Linda twice since our last meeting, and each time has spoken words of encouragement and given advice that has been very helpful to the Board in finding its way out of difficulty."[10]

Then he quoted Ellen White based on a recent talk she had given: "Never are we to utter a word that would arouse doubt or fear, or that would cast shadows over the minds of others. . . . When I hear criticism and complaint, or an expression of doubt or fear, I know that he who thus speaks has his eyes turned away from the Saviour. . . . Let us not look on the dark side. As soon as we yield to the temptation to do this, we shall have plenty of company. But there is nothing to be gained by looking on the dark side."[11]

### CME's Report Card

The mounting pressure prompted Irwin to make a powerful appeal: "How to provide the proper agencies and facilities to entitle us to a proper rating and classification in the American Medical Association is the greatest problem confronting this meeting. To insure the success of this school as a medical college, will demand quick and imperative action upon the part of the Constituency and Board of Management."[12]

Irwin then explained the system of four ratings adopted by the American Medical Association. He pointed out that various state associations were already accepting these measurements:

**Class A+ Colleges.** Acceptable.

**Class A Colleges.** Need to improve in certain respects, but are otherwise acceptable.

**Class B Colleges.** If general improvements are made, they might be made acceptable.

**Class C Colleges.** Requires a complete reorganization to make them acceptable.

So, where did CME stand? "Our school," the General Conference president admitted, "is placed in the list of colleges rated Class C."[13]

To further emphasize the gravity of CME's situation, Irwin reported that Abbott had received notice from the Maryland Medical Association stating that students from C-rated colleges would be excluded from taking their state board examinations. Moreover, a recent letter from Colwell said that 25 or more of the state boards had made the same ruling. In fact, the probability existed that *all* state boards would take the same action in the near future. In the face of this peril, some action had to be taken to insure a better rating. "[Otherwise] we will be compelled to abandon our efforts to graduate physicians who will be allowed to practice in harmony with the laws of our country."[14]

To complicate matters further, CME had suffered heavy financial losses and many difficulties in raising funds. On the other hand, the sanitarium was experiencing major growth. Its patronage and its earnings had reached an all-time high. Thus, the General Conference appointed a committee of "brethren" to look at expenses and to recommend changes in the methods of operation at the sanitarium.

Speaking about the challenges with CME, Irwin said, "While we have come to a crisis in this work, we are not discouraged or disheartened in the least." He reminded the constituency that Ellen White had advised them *not* to exhibit doubt and fear, nor to look on the dark side. "What we want is courage in the Lord, and then we shall by His help and blessing make of Loma Linda just what God designs it should be."[15]

All of this distress notwithstanding, Ruble reported that student confidence and morale remained high. Actually, most students had returned, and they were determined to make the school a success.

"In spite of the fact that there was no active progress being made in providing further necessary facilities for clinical experience, the students have been kept satisfied with the promise that these would be provided at the earliest possible date. . . . We feel on the whole that we are making all the progress that could be expected with the handicap under which we are laboring of not having hospital facilities sufficient for the giving of a proper education to our students."[16]

Although the San Bernardino County Hospital had made some clinical facilities available to the students, opportunities were limited to two medical wards three days a week for two hours. Political influences prevented any privileges in the hospital's surgical clinics. These were just stopgap measures, not a real solution. CME appealed to the San Bernardino County board of supervisors, attempting to improve upon the agreement. Unfortunately, even after the meeting diagnostic experience was still limited, and the medical superintendent fully controlled patient management and the administration of treatments, which differed greatly from the denominationally unique hydrotherapy treatments that CME wished to demonstrate to its students.

Once again, Ruble emphasized the need for CME to have its own hospital. Only then could denominational principles (as practiced in the sanitariums) be taught:

"There is no way of teaching physiological therapeutics without having a goodly number of patients upon whom to demonstrate. . . . The last two years of our medical course are the most important years because they are the years when the principles of healthful living and physiological therapeutics are emphasized and taught in detail. . . . If we had access to all the county hospitals in California this would not at all suffice for giving the education which must be imparted to our students.

"The question of the continuance of our medical school must be met fairly and squarely at this time. A medical school must be chartered under existing laws which are based upon certain definite requirements for imparting a medical education. These laws dictate and supervise the course of study, the efficiency of the faculty, laboratory equipment, library advantages, hospital facilities, and the dispensary advantages that must be provided."[17]

Ironically, the previous year's accreditation survey of laboratory courses for the first two years had actually been good. The school could have received a class B ranking for its courses; however, CME had identified itself as providing a complete course. And it lacked at least half of the facilities needed—a hospital and outpatient dispensary. Inevitably, the survey documented its deficiencies. Meeting the crisis head-on, Ruble *confronted* the board. The urgency of the matter had driven him to the edge, and he stated the case in the *strongest* words possible.

"This means death to our college unless immediate steps are taken to provide what is necessary for giving a thorough medical course. One year has already passed since this matter was placed before this board, and what we see today was fully prophesied at that time. The question now before us is, Are we to make good in establishing this medical college? If so the hospital must be built at once."[18]

Ruble reiterated the immediate necessity of providing dispensary facilities for the school: "With these two most important features provided, in addition to what we have, there is no reason why our school should not be rated sufficiently high to admit our students to any of the state examining boards when they have completed their course."[19]

## Making Do With Little

Meanwhile, CME's administrators had not been idle, Ruble assured the board. They were doing all they could with limited resources. They had opened a temporary treatment facility on Monday, October 28, 1912. The southwest cottage on the east crest of the hill could accommodate up to ten patients in its eight rooms. One room was used as an office and one for examinations, dressings, and clinics.

The effort proved to be convincing. The very next day, January 28, 1913, the constituency finally acknowledged the need for a permanent hospital: "We hereby approve of the plan of the Hospital . . . and authorize its construction at a cost not to exceed $20,000, including furnishings, and recommend that the Board arrange at once for the extensive solicitation of gifts for the erection of the building, and that this work be carried on by solicitors appointed by the Board."

Now, there was nothing left to do but find the money! The board requested that the General Conference Committee appoint a Sabbath offering as early as possible in an effort to collect liberal donations. [20]

[1]George A. Irwin, president of the board of trustees, special meeting of the constituency of the College of Medical Evangelists, "Report by Elder G. A. Irwin," minutes, January 27, 1913, p. 10.

[2]Carrol S. Small, M.D., "A Hospital? When We Already Have a Sanitarium?" *Diamond Memories*, Loma Linda, California, Alumni Association, School of Medicine of Loma Linda University, 1984, p. 27.

[3]CME constituency meeting, minutes, 1912, p. 13.

[4]CME board of trustees, minutes, March 27, 1912, pp. 65, 66.

[5]*Ibid.*, March 27, 1912, pp. 75, 76.

[6]*Ibid.*, pp. 79, 80.

[7]College president's council, minutes, June 1-6, 1912, p. 214.

[8]CME board of trustees, minutes, December 4, 1912, pp. 125, 126.

[9]CME constituency meeting, minutes, January 27, 1913, pp. 129, 130.

[10]CME constituency meeting, minutes, January 27, 1913, p. 78.

[11]*Ibid.*, January 27, 1913, p. 78; Ellen G. White, quoted from November 9, 1912, meeting of the CME board of trustees.

[12]*Ibid.*, January 27, 1913, p. 84.

[13]*Ibid.*, January 27, 1913, p. 138.

[14]*Ibid.*

[15]*Ibid.*, pp. 141, 142.

[16]*Ibid.*, pp. 142, 143.

[17]*Ibid.*, p. 145.

[18]*Ibid.*, p. 147.

[19]*Ibid.*, p. 148.

[20]*Ibid.*, pp. 167, 168.

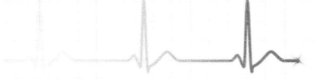

# Chapter 3

# What Are Our Alternatives?

C ME continued exploring all clinical experience options for its student physicians. At the board meeting in March 1913 a question arose for the first time, a question that would be subject to months of heated debate. Could opening a dispensary (outpatient clinic) in Los Angeles help with CME's clinical training requirements?

To this end a committee was formed to determine the possibility and costs associated with operating a dispensary in Los Angeles.[1] They also voted to ask the Sanitarium Association of Seventh-day Adventists of Southern California to allow CME students to use its institutions.

### Improved Educational Standards

The board's efforts to increase educational opportunities at CME complemented other adjustments to improve the institution's educational standards. The board stepped up the prerequisites for admission. Prospective students now had to complete at least 14 grades or their equivalent, including one year of college studies in physics, chemistry, and biology. Students also had to possess a reading knowledge of at least one modern language besides English (preferably German or French). The new requirements went into effect on January 1, 1915. These prerequisites had to be obtained at Pacific Union College, Walla Walla College, Union College, Emmanuel Missionary College, Mt. Vernon College, or South Lancaster Academy. Also, these students would be required to earn a bachelor's degree before graduation.[2]

CME's most urgent need prompted the board to send Ruble and Abbott on a mission the next day. They were to return to San Bernardino County Hospital and ascertain what *additional* clinical privileges might be arranged there for Loma Linda students.[3]

## The Los Angeles Dispensary

Still struggling with its lack of outpatient facilities, the board voted on August 16, 1913, to appoint a committee of three members to locate and open a dispensary in Los Angeles.[4] "We have completed arrangements for a dispensary in Los Angeles," Ruble wrote to Dr. Edward H. Risley on September 12, 1913. "We are told by the Health Officers, the Nursing Commission, and the Board of Charities [that this property] is the very best location in the city." Situated near the Santa Fe railway station, it was 27 feet by 63 feet. In order to make the dispensary a free clinic, the city of Los Angeles proposed to furnish all the supplies and provide a nurse.[5]

Ruble said that the fifth-year class would spend most of the year in Los Angeles, and the fourth-year class might be there the latter third of the year. "I have . . . made arrangements for our students to attend all of the clinics they are offering in the [Los Angeles] County Hospital. They are to have the same privileges as other students of medical schools in the city and you know they receive most of their clinical experience in the County Hospital there. Our students will be admitted to all surgical and medical clinics, and will have the advantage of the teaching from the best instructors who hold clinics there. I feel, myself, that we have advantages superior to the other schools to offer to our students, and there is no doubt but what we shall get better recognition when the time comes for another investigation."[6]

All of this was good, but . . . at best, it was a makeshift arrangement to substitute for a large teaching hospital. To emphasize increasing concerns over the monumental task of funding CME, the board voted once again to seek broad support from the church.

## A Big Mistake?

Over the months, the financial deficits of the institution became increasingly apparent and painful. Some board members questioned whether the denomination should have undertaken the founding of a medical school at all. The first comment questioning the future of CME appears in the board minutes from October 22, 1913: "Elder Knox felt that our finances are now beyond the grasp of the denomination; and asked, What is the future of Loma Linda?" Even Daniells voiced doubt. Had the CME board made a mistake in establishing a full medical school when the institution was successfully conducting a medical missionary school?[7] Although enormous effort had been expended, the returns had been poor. Depression set in and everything seemed to go in reverse.

A major cutback was in the offing. These discouraging words led to a serious evaluation of CME's curriculum in an effort to reduce expenses. A few days later, after much discussion, the board compared the costs of running a three-year school ($10,000) with the expenses of running a five-year school ($19,020). This figure estimated the expenses of operating a 70-bed hospital. Acknowledging the reality of their financial difficulty, the board voted to drop the fourth and fifth year of the medical course. [8]

But before the board implemented this drastic decision, a storm of protest erupted. Dr. Daniel Kress acknowledged the practicality of a three-year medical missionary course. However, Elder F. M. Wilcox felt that instruction from Ellen White called for a full medical course, and Elder W. C. White thought that the church's young people should benefit from a full course of study. Ruble spoke of the openings in Los Angeles for fifth-year medical students, and Dr. David Paulson recalled "the rocks in the stream" that were met by the American Medical Missionary College in Battle Creek, Michigan.[9] The next day, the board established a commission to investigate the implications and differences between a three- and five-year medical curriculum.

## The Loma Linda Hospital

At this same time, the new hospital, located in the middle of what is now the basic sciences quadrangle, neared completion. Fortunately, at the moment, no one could foresee the disappointment it would cause.

On November 24, 1913, Burden told the board that the estimated cost of running the new facility was entirely too high. Others agreed. The chair suggested that all possible information concerning the cost of operating the hospital be presented at the March 1914 constituency meeting.[10]

Nonetheless, that same day, board members named the new facility Loma Linda Hospital. They made it available for sanitarium patients and school

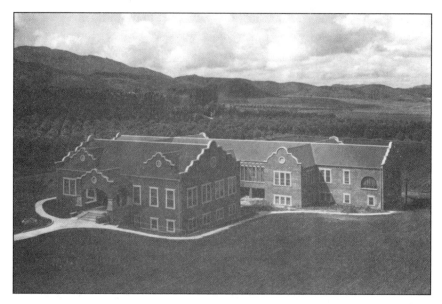

The first Loma Linda Hospital (1913)

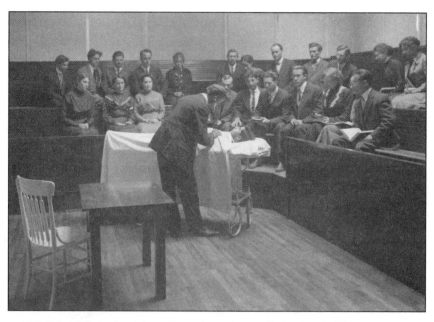

Archie W. Truman, M.D., teaches a class of first- and second-year medical students in 1914.

clinics, and placed it under the medical supervision of Ruble. Patients would be moved into the new hospital on December 1, 1913.[11]

## The Debate Goes On: Five or Three?

By the March 1914 constituency meeting the issue of reducing the five-year curriculum to three still had not been resolved. The Washington Council had met in the fall of 1913, but E. E. Andross reported that no decision had been made, because the council said that the matter was for the constituency to decide. A committee had been appointed to investigate and prepare a report, but it had failed to meet, so the philosophical debate raged on. (What caused this lapse in reporting is not recorded.)

Once more, the chair repeated his question as to whether or not the five-year course should continue: "Are medical men needed in this message? Is the Lord calling for such a school as we have been trying to carry? When we know for what the Lord is calling, we will know better how to work to attain that end."[12] He added that there was a real "scarcity of medical men who supported principles of truth."

Committee members expressed many divergent views—some drawn from previous discussions. Dr. T. J. Evans admitted surprise that the denomination had as many faithful physicians as it had, considering the error that was woven into worldly education. He reiterated the fact that the time had come when the church's young people should be educated in their own schools. He suggested that self-supporting physicians might be recruited who would be able to give some time to CME's educational program in Los Angeles.

Dr. W. A. George said he thought the matter of the church having its own medical school already had been settled! Of course we should have a medical school. The only question for him was how and where it should be conducted.

W. C. White expressed thankfulness for the faithful work done by those who "have been on the ground." He acknowledged tremendous difficulties and expressed strong support of the full five-year course. Anything less, he said, would deprive the school of the power it should wield. He feared that a shortened course would force the most valuable young people to obtain their training in worldly schools, and eventually be lost to the work of the church.

W. A. Spicer wondered how the AMA would regard the school if it succeeded in gaining privileges at the Los Angeles County Hospital.

Ruble stated that the superintendent of the county hospital supported the work of CME and that all he needed was the permission of the board of supervisors to proceed. The new Loma Linda Hospital, he said, would provide students with "a training in therapeutics such as we hold as a denomination."

The result? The constituency voted to appoint a committee of five to study the question further. More stalling and more delay.

The General Conference Commission, however, did ascertain what recognition might be granted to CME if it conducted the fourth and fifth years in Los Angeles, and they delivered this report to the constituency meeting. The board then reversed itself and voted to offer the first three years at Loma Linda and continue the fourth and fifth years in Los Angeles.[13]

During the same constituency meeting Ruble delivered an encouraging report:

"With the completion of this year we will have demonstrated the possibility of conducting a full medical course in the denomination. There has been the best spirit of cooperation in the school during the year that has existed since the medical school was started. Very little discipline has been called for in any way. The students are generally taking a deep interest in bringing the school up to the high standard it should occupy."[14]

Most people today do not realize the gravity of the circumstances that Loma Linda repeatedly faced. The thread runs throughout the history of the institution. Any one of the crises could have totally derailed CME.

## The Loma Linda Hospital and Its Destiny

Regarding the new hospital, Ruble rejoiced in the fact that it "is possible for our students to have under their own supervision different diseases which they may treat according to the system of physiologic therapeutics which have been accepted by this denomination." So far, so good.

Hospital patients, however, numbered 15 to 20. No great effort was made to fill the hospital "on account of the desirability of conducting this part of our institution on as nearly a self-supporting basis as is possible." CME endowed several beds to receive worthy cases that would be of great teaching value.[15]

In an editorial in *The Medical Evangelist* during the spring of 1914, Ruble reported recent progress at CME, including completion of the new hospital and the graduation of the first class of physicians:

"The present school year thus far has been the most prosperous and encouraging in the history of the College of Medical Evangelists. For four years the College has been building first with one class, then two, and so on until the present year finds five classes, or the entire course in progress. This seems good to those who have toiled and prayed for the success of the school, for we feel that we are now on the home stretch.

"At the last General Conference sufficient means was contributed to construct a new hospital for the use of the College. This has been completed and is now in use. The Hospital is a great asset to the school. About twenty patients have been in constant attendance for the past three or four months."[16]

Ruble reported that students were gaining clinical experience in the new hospital, the sanitarium, the San Bernardino County Hospital, the Los Angeles County Hospital, and at the dispensary in Los Angeles, "all of which is very valuable."

Still, a dark secret lurked just beneath the surface: The new 70-bed hospital did not meet expectations. Financial stringency made it impossible to operate it as a charity institution, and there were not enough paying patients to fill the beds. Therefore the facility failed to provide an adequate number of patients for clinical education. Situated in a rural valley, it did not provide the breadth of clinical experience needed for the training of physicians.[17]

For whatever reason, the commission referred to the patients in the new hospital as "inmates." Sadly, during the months of January and February in 1914 the number of inmates averaged only 15, including babies. The next discussion focused on how the building should now be used. Opinions differed widely, but all agreed that "it cannot be used for the clinical work of the college as was first thought necessary for the profit of the school."

Some suggested completing the basement and constructing a dining room and kitchen facilities for helpers and hospital patients. Another idea involved creating treatment rooms that could be used in connection with the sanitarium. Members of the constituency meeting did "not feel competent" to make the decision. They agreed only that the building "cannot be used as originally designed for the college clinical hospital."[18]

Dr. Carrol S. Small (class of 1934) later penned perhaps the most colorful description of the demise of the first Loma Linda Hospital: "So the hospital went out, not with a bang, but a whimper. How sad! All that sweat and tears and epinephrine [adrenaline, a hormone] and prayers and cries, and—pffft! All eyes now turned to Los Angeles."[19]

Even though the Loma Linda Hospital continued in operation until clinical resources in Los Angeles could be expanded, the commission report of March 25, 1914, concluded:

"It is now conceded by all connected with the college that the clinical work, or most of it will have to be done in Los Angeles, utilizing the dispensary, and making such hospital arrangements as may be possible and acceptable to the governing medical board."[20]

### The Los Angeles Solution

The most obvious location to provide clinical experience for CME students was the Los Angeles County Hospital. It had become available two days a week and offered excellent clinical training, especially in surgery. When CME administrators requested teaching privileges, some physicians had no interest. They felt that too few students were not worth the bother. Others, however, were more charitable and supported the request. Thus, a working relationship developed.[21]

Prospects were good that outpatient medical clinics there would provide further educational opportunities. The Glendale Sanitarium had offered exceptional medical and surgical privileges. Ruble also spoke of another innovation with "unlimited opportunities." That is, outpatient practice in the homes of the people where "the line of therapeutics which we have adopted in our institution" could be used.[22]

Based on these factors, a new schedule went into effect. Students spent three and a half years studying basic sciences in Loma Linda, where they also received practical experience in the sanitarium and hospital. They spent the next full year gaining clinical experience in Los Angeles, and then they spent the remaining six months of their education reviewing and taking examinations at Loma Linda.[23]

The first CME graduates had to step forward to claim their rights. Shortly after the six physicians graduated on June 11, 1914, they applied to be admitted for the State Board of Medical Examiners of California examinations. Only if they passed the examination could they qualify for a license to practice medicine and surgery in California. Although they applied in time, they failed to receive a reply.

Knowing the time and place in Los Angeles where the exams were to be administered, the Loma Linda graduates boldly presented themselves as candidates. Surprised and perplexed, the state officials didn't know what to do with the unexpected arrivals. The CME graduates told the officials that they were qualified to sit for the exams and wondered why their applications had not received attention. They appeared, they said, because they had not been denied. Also, they felt prepared.

As officials tried to decide what to do, the time for testing to start came and went, causing the candidates from the University of Southern California to complain about the delay. Finally, officials decided, on the spot, to admit the CME Class of 1914. Fortunately, each graduate did very well.[24]

### Providence Provides a Man for the Hour

Meanwhile, on the other side of the continent, God had worked behind the scenes in Madison, Tennessee. There would be a man to meet the legal, financial, and political challenges of CME's future—Percy T. Magan. A middle-aged minister/teacher, Magan had a close friend and colleague, Edward A. Sutherland. In 1910 the latter tried to persuade Magan to join him in becoming a physician.

After much soul-searching and discussion (including counsel from Ellen White), the two men decided to attend medical school together at the University of Tennessee Medical School. Ellen White had said that if they would go to Nashville and take the medical course, "The Lord will raise you up friends." At the time, these men did not understand the importance of the instruction. Later, after Magan had become associated with CME, this statement was fulfilled to the letter. Men with whom Magan had been associated as teachers in Nashville and Memphis, Tennessee, proved to be real friends in opening the way to solve some of the most difficult problems at CME.[25] Both legends in education, Magan and Sutherland became physicians on June 6, 1914, thus continuing their 28-year professional partnership.[26]

### "Educating" Ellen White

Although Sutherland found fault with his medical education in Tennessee, he did not criticize the medical profession itself. Having strong feelings about his personal experience, he told Magan that he had decided to share his insights and wisdom about medical education with Ellen White. "I'm going out and have a talk with Sister White. I'm going to tell Sister White some things that undoubtedly she doesn't know anything about in running a medical school."[27]

This statement illustrates Sutherland's recognition of Ellen White's continuing prominence in developing the school of medicine in Loma Linda. At the same time, he was acknowledging the sorry state of medical education in America. But the times were changing. The Abraham Flexner Report, sponsored by the Carnegie Foundation for the Advancement of Teaching, intended to improve the quality of medical education in America.

In light of this report and the new standards for medical training Sutherland sincerely felt that it would be impossible for the church to develop an acceptable school of medicine. The high standards would surely be insurmountable. He told Ellen White that developing an approved medical school in Loma Linda simply couldn't be done. CME didn't have the money to put up the necessary buildings. This fact had been demonstrated the previous year when CME tried to build its first hospital in Loma Linda. Furthermore, it didn't have a competent faculty, and it couldn't get one. Therefore, Loma Linda could not possibly succeed.

Every time Sutherland shared his concerns and ideas about what it would take to belong to the American Medical Association, Ellen White responded according to her providential insights. She stated that the Lord had shown her that the College of Medical Evangelists would become one of the finest schools of medicine in the land. She insisted that CME's graduates would someday make the best physicians. Indeed, they would go to the ends of the earth.

Still, Sutherland wouldn't give up. "Then I would get my breath and I'd meet her again the next day and I'd start to tell her something new, try to go over the same thing that I did in a more impressive way, but I never got anywhere."

Ellen White held her ground, always giving the same response—CME was going to be a success; the Lord had "planted it," and He would make it one of the strongest institutions in the world. Sutherland recounted his frustrating conversations to Magan.[28] He had to admit, however, that he had more than met his match in Ellen White.

### Dr. Newton Evans, CME's New President

In August 1914 CME elected Dr. Newton G. Evans to be Loma Linda's new president. Previously, he had been the medical superintendent of the

Madison Sanitarium and professor of pathology at the University of Tennessee. (Ruble had asked to be relieved of his administrative responsibilities.)

Just after Newton Evans arrived, Colwell again inspected CME, including its Los Angeles dispensary. Although encouraged by Colwell's evaluation, Evans felt he needed assistance in attaining a higher accreditation rating for the institution. The report card still read "C." The new president immediately remembered Magan, one of his educational colleagues at Madison, Tennessee. In fact, it was Newton Evans who had encouraged him to become a physician.

Magan was now a recognized diagnostician, a loyal church member, and an astute educator. With his support, the Madison institution supported Loma Linda with leaders and financial assistance. Because of Magan's tenacious but winning ways, he would become instrumental in representing the church-related institution to the American Medical Association.

On January 20, 1915, the board voted to send Evans, Magan, and Ruble to represent CME to the Council on Medical Education of the American Medical Association. (Although not yet officially connected with CME, Magan started forming friendships in the political circles of the AMA when it met in Chicago in February 1915. These connections eventually became extremely valuable in future contacts.)

In the meantime, in order to focus more denominational attention on CME, the board voted on January 30, 1915, to invite the North American Division Conference to hold its medical convention in Loma Linda from March 19 to 23.

### The Presidential Report for 1915

One day after the medical convention, Newton Evans delivered the president's report at CME's constituency meeting.[29] The topics were definitely not new ones.

- **Enrollment** – The number of students who entered the first year of medical school that year was much smaller than any of the first-year classes in the past.
- **Entrance requirements** – The requirements to begin medical school had increased, which could have contributed to the reduced class size. Applicants now had to have completed one year of regular college work in addition to the twelve grades of academic work.

- **Faculty** – The number of instructors now numbered 56—20 in Loma Linda, 13 in Los Angeles, and the rest serving as special lecturers. Because the CME faculty had arranged its medical school curriculum to span five years, each student spent four years at Loma Linda and the fifth year in Los Angeles. This schedule made it necessary to have teachers in Loma Linda and in Los Angeles.
- **Clinical division** – This division remained woefully inadequate. Teaching privileges continued only by special arrangements with physicians who had regular appointments on the clinical staff at the Los Angeles County Hospital. The 28 patients a day treated at CME's Los Angeles outpatient dispensary did not meet the requirements of the Council on Medical Education, which called for 100 patients. Evans referred to the San Bernardino County Hospital with high hopes. Recent plans to increase the size of that hospital would improve the clinical opportunities for CME students. The expanded facility had an average daily census of 150 patients, and future plans had been made to build a new $150,000 hospital.
- **Loma Linda Hospital** – Designed to serve 70 patients, the hospital accommodated only 12 to 26. Evans advised that CME should make "strong efforts to fill this hospital with patients." So far, that hadn't happened. After such great effort, CME still didn't have a satisfactory arrangement for clinical training.

Courageously Newton Evans tried to end on a positive note. CME had well-equipped laboratories that complemented a good working library of more than 10,000 volumes, including scientific medical journals: "We feel that the school has been making definite progress in all lines. There is a feeling of unity and enthusiasm on the part of all the teachers and an improvement in the spiritual condition and consecration of the student body is evident."

He finally appealed for a strengthening of CME by building up the work of the new Loma Linda Hospital and adding teachers to the laboratory staff. He indicated that at least one year of clinical teaching should be provided at Loma Linda, and that the Loma Linda teaching faculty needed to be strengthened significantly.[30]

### Still *Not Enough*

CME had to move beyond the dream. It had to have its own hospital in

Los Angeles. Newton Evans challenged the constituency to provide enlarged dispensary facilities in Los Angeles. That, however, would be only the beginning. He declared unequivocally that CME must have a hospital of its own in connection with and in close proximity to the dispensary.

News of the Loma Linda Sanitarium provided a welcome balance and encouragement. T. J. Evans, superintendent of the Loma Linda Sanitarium, offered a positive report on patient admissions and the significant financial benefits that had resulted:

"God has blessed us with a regular patronage which has been the best in the history of the institution during the summer months. This has supplied a greater financial income for our work. Previous to this time our patronage was so low and our expenses were so great that we suffered severe financial loss each summer, but at no time during this summer has our patronage [at both the sanitarium and hospital] been below 52, and it has averaged 69. Our average this year has been something like 20 better than the year previous, for the same period of time."[31]

On June 17, 1915, the board made a truly far-reaching decision. They decided to ask the North American Division to build the "Ellen G. White Memorial Hospital" at a cost not to exceed $50,000. They would also solicit cooperation from people who could provide property suitable for a home for medical students. The entire plan would be submitted for approval at the church's Autumn Council.[32] This decision came just four weeks before Ellen White died on July 16, 1915.

### More Curriculum Changes

At the November constituency meeting, Newton Evans announced a radical change in the medical school curriculum. CME would now provide a four-year medical course of 36 weeks. Entrance requirements had been increased from one year to two years of college studies, in addition to twelve grades of schoolwork. "The two years of college studies must include certain specified subjects; namely, chemistry, physics, biology, and the study of some modern language in addition to English."[33] (This action was an amplification of the vote first taken in 1913.)

Evans reported that medical students received two and a half years of clinical experience in Loma Linda, San Bernardino, and Los Angeles, "practically one year of this time being spent in Los Angeles." The Los Angeles dispensary now saw 30 to 40 patients a day. The 1,200-bed Los Angeles County Hospital on Mission Road, overseen by volunteer members of the hospital staff, provided both inpatient and outpatient experience.

The number of patients at the Loma Linda Hospital had increased to an average of 30 patients a day, most of them available for clinical teaching. Evans expected patronage to increase to its capacity of 70.[34]

Nine of the 12 graduates from the second class took the California State Board examinations in July of 1915, and all passed successfully. "Since it is true that the legal standing of the graduates of the school depends upon the standing of the school, and that the standing of the school to a certain extent is influenced by the success of these graduates in their examinations before State Boards, it is a source of much gratitude that so many of these recent graduates were successful."[35]

CME's great need for more acceptable clinical facilities in Los Angeles concluded the report, but one promising development regarding CME's standing with the AMA remained to be told. It had to do with the report card grade.

"We have recently received word from Colwell, of the Council on Medical Education, that he expects to visit the school again this fall or winter, and that he hopes to find conditions so improved, especially along clinical lines, that he can recommend a higher rating for the school by the Council on Medical Education.

"It may be of interest to know that Dr. Malloney, who is vice president of the California State Board of Medical Examiners, recently wrote to Colwell, strongly urging that a change in the rating of the College of Medical Evangelists should be made by the Council on Medical Education, and insisting that the present rating is an injustice to our school."

The fact that influential members of the California State Board of Medical Examiners (without solicitation) had noticed Loma Linda was cause for rejoicing. Surely they would see some progress in CME's work. The "instruction from the Lord" had led Loma Linda to believe that legal recognition would be "in the line of His Providence."[36]

As it would turn out, they were not yet "home free." Not quite yet.

[1] CME board of trustees, minutes, March 26, 1913, p. 3. Committee members: Dr. Ruble, John Burden, Dr. Daniel D. Comstock, H. W. Lindsay, and F. M. Burg.

[2] *Ibid.*, March 27, 1913, pp. 7, 8.

[3] *Ibid.*, p. 6.

[4] *Ibid.*, August 16, 1913, p. 2. Committee members: George K. Abbott, W. D. Salisbury, Daniel D. Comstock.

[5] *The Medical Evangelist,* June 1959, p. 23.

[6] *Ibid.*

[7] CME board of trustees, minutes, October 22, 1913, p. 3.

[8] *Ibid.*, October 26, 1913, p. 1.

[9] *Ibid.*, p. 4.

[10] *Ibid.*, October 31, 1913, p. 1.

[11] *Ibid.*, November 24, 1913, p. 3.

[12] CME constituency meeting, minutes, March 25, 1914, pp. 37, 39.

[13] *Ibid.*, pp. 37, 39-40, 42-43, 73.

[14] *Ibid.*, pp. 37-39.

[15] *Ibid.*

[16] *The Medical Evangelist,* first quarter, 1914, p. 10.

[17] *Ibid.*, November 1953, p. 9; Clarence A. Miller, "The Loma Linda San," *Diamond Memories*, p. 21.

[18] CME constituency meeting, minutes, March 25, 1914, p. 210.

[19] Carrol Small, M.D., "A Hospital? When We Already Have a Sanitarium?" *Diamond Memories*, p. 29.

[20] CME constituency meeting, minutes, March 25, 1914, p. 211 (of big book).

[21] Walter E. Macpherson, M.D., "The County," *Diamond Memories*, p. 76.

[22] CME constituency meeting, minutes, March 25, 1914, p. 11.

[23] *Ibid.*, p. 8.

[24] William Wagner, M.D, letter to Richard A Schaefer, September 2003, reporting a personal discussion with Fred E. Herzer, M.D., CME class of 1914.

[25] Edward A. Sutherland, M.D., *Chronological Arrangement of Events in the Life of Percy Tilson Magan and Those Associated With Him*, 1949, p. 17.

[26] Merlin L. Neff, "Things Medical," *For God and CME*, pp. 152, 154. Among the projects that Magan and Sutherland shared was the moving of Battle Creek College to Berrien Springs, Michigan, where it was renamed "Emmanuel Missionary College" (now Andrews University). The two men cofounded the "Nashville Agricultural and Normal Institute," later to become Madison College.

[27] Department of Archives and Special Collections, Loma Linda University, document file 3229.06.

[28] *Ibid.*

[29] CME constituency meeting, minutes, March 24, 1915, pp. 3-7.

[30] *Ibid.*, pp. 7, 8.

[31] *Ibid.*, pp. 7-11.

[32] CME board of trustees, minutes, June 17, 1915, p. 2.

[33] *Ibid.*, November 11, 1915, pp. 2, 3.

[34] *Ibid.*, March 28, 1915, p. 228.

[35] *Ibid.*, p. 233.

[36] *Ibid.*, pp. 234, 235.

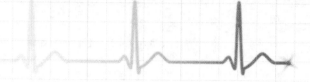

Chapter 4:

# CME at a Crossroads

By 1915 people began to question whether CME's growing pains would ever go away. The American Medical Association kept rating the college at a substandard status, and, moreover, the supporting Seventh-day Adventist Church lived under the shadow of an ever-growing debt.

These dire considerations motivated the church to hold its 1915 Autumn Council in Loma Linda. CME accommodated 150 delegates in a tent city erected near the future site of the Centennial Complex. High on the agenda was the determination to exercise fiscal responsibility. The council adopted a firm resolution to reduce church indebtedness; this was an understandable but ominous action as far as Loma Linda was concerned! By this time CME had accumulated an astronomical $400,000 in debt. In those days such a situation caused the church to experience one massive shudder of apprehension.[1]

### What Shall We Do With the School of Medicine?

Funding was the main question that dominated the meetings, as well as many more that had been held before. The church appointed a subcommittee to study the crisis. The subcommittee came up with only two solutions: call home a large number of foreign missionaries and divert their mission subsidy to Loma Linda, or close the college.

Since the subcommittee members considered diverting mission funds to the college to be unthinkable, they recommended closing the School of Medicine. A painful, almost paralyzing silence engulfed the council room. Then an old, gray-haired brother arose from the front. In a quavering voice, he declared:

"Brethren, I am bewildered. I can hardly believe my eyes and my ears. What is this I hear you say? We must close this school? . . . Soon the vote will be taken, but before it is taken, let me say this:

"You know who I am, George I. Butler. I used to be president of the General Conference, and I think I received more testimonies from the servant of the Lord than any of you, and most of them rebuked me. We were at times urged to do what seemed impossible, but when we went forward by faith, the way opened. Brethren, I believe in God and in His prophets!"

Waving a pamphlet containing Ellen White's instructions to establish and operate a medical college in California, Butler appealed earnestly for faith and confidence in the divine counsels. Then he added stoutly: "Now, Brother Daniells [president of the General Conference] will soon call for a vote. When he does, here is one old hand that will not go up." Butler held out his shaking arm: "This hand has not learned how to vote to close what God says should be open."

One of the delegates, A. V. Olsen, wrote years later, "I thrust my right hand into my pocket and said to myself: 'I know another hand that will not go up!'"[2]

Some felt strongly that the church should no longer attempt the impossible and should close CME. Others suggested that the curriculum should be reduced to the first two years of basic sciences. Students would then be encouraged to complete their medical education elsewhere. Burden and Magan felt strongly that the recently adjusted four-year school of medicine curriculum should remain intact. Most delegates favored the two-year plan. Feelings ran deep. In a metaphor attributed to Ellen White, Magan compared the conflict and resolution to a "battle to be followed by a march."[3]

Ellen White's views on Loma Linda went back a very long way and were "the gold standard" against which all debate had to be measured. Even before CME had been incorporated, she insisted that the youth of the church should not be forced to attend medical schools that might compromise their beliefs and ideals. Approximately six years earlier, Ellen White had told Burden in an interview about her feelings on the subject: "I felt a heavy burden this morning, when I read over a letter that I found in my room, in which a plan was outlined for having medical students take some work at Loma Linda, but to get the finishing touches of their education from some worldly institution. God forbid that such a plan should be followed."[4]

A few days later, she reiterated her position in a letter to Burden: "Some have advised that students should, after taking some work at Loma Linda, complete their medical education in worldly colleges. But this is not in harmony with the Lord's plan."[5]

Whether Burden reported these statements, and whether they impacted the meeting, is not recorded.

### Woman Power Arrives

As the heated discussions about the fate of CME continued, a new and surprising source of support appeared. Four nondelegate women asked to be heard by the council. The group included Dr. Florence Keller, a pioneer physician in New Zealand; Josephine Gotzian, a wealthy widow; Mrs. Stephen N. Haskell, a woman of faith and strong belief; and her sister, Emma Gray.

They urged the council to continue the school and suggested that the women of the denomination raise the funds with which to build the needed hospital for clinical teaching in Los Angeles. Moreover, they felt that the hospital should be named after Ellen G. White, who had died just four months earlier. The delegation of women was, indeed, extraordinary. Later, Magan remembered that a "sacred hush pervaded the room."[6]

Inspired, no doubt, by the women's proposal, Daniells made a powerful speech the very next day. With alarm, he reviewed Ellen White's position on Loma Linda:

"My brethren, I am astounded and I must speak. If I do not say my mind I will be a coward and unworthy of your confidence. Brethren, listen to me. We all profess faith in the Spirit of Prophecy, but we forget that one of the last things the prophet ever wrote was that our young men and women should be given their full training in our own school and should not be forced to go to worldly schools. And here we are, before the prophet is hardly cold in her grave, proposing that our young men and women shall only have half of their education from us and then shall be turned loose in these worldly schools. Now, I protest against it. That is all I can do, but I do most earnestly protest it. We can build up this school. We can support it. We can do anything God wants us to do."[7]

Earlier, Newton Evans had invited Magan to attend the council meetings. He well knew that Magan's interests, leadership talents, and enthusiasm would complement CME's administration.[8] Near the close of the discussions, Magan, an acknowledged orator, found that he could not contain himself any longer. (What would you expect from such an extroverted Irishman?) According to Sutherland, he made a most wonderful and eloquent plea for the college to continue as a four-year school.

When he saw how close this institution was to being closed up, the spirit of the Lord moved upon him, and he let everything out that he could put out to show that it would be practically impossible, at least impractical, to try to educate trained doctors by the method that they would have to pursue if they didn't have their own college.[9]

From personal experience Magan knew exactly what Adventist medical students would face. "His words were so pointed and took such a deep hold that men who strongly opposed the continuance of the school were practically unable to answer Magan's arguments, and those who were battling for the school took a new grip."[10]

When the council voted, everyone voted to keep the school open. According to Magan, "There had been another battle; there would now be another march."[11] The church authorized CME to operate a full-fledged, four-year curriculum. The school would teach basic sciences in Loma Linda and provide clinical education in Los Angeles at the proposed $61,000 White Memorial Hospital. The denomination did not recall any foreign missionaries or divert foreign mission offerings to Loma Linda.

That night Newton Evans confronted Magan. "Now, Percy, you saved the College tonight, and you've got to come over here and help run it." According to Sutherland, Evans had Magan right where he could do nothing but surrender. And surrender he did. Magan's acceptance thrilled Evans. The two would become a most effective team—Magan excelled at fund-raising and Evans possessed the educational vision.[12]

Historian Keld J. Reynolds remarked on the way "the scent of battle pleased the fighting Irishman."[13] In a letter to Dr. David Paulson immediately following the council, Magan summarized the battle as one of the fiercest contests he had ever witnessed. Indeed, "if the Lord had not worked some miracles there would have been a terrible state of affairs." He acknowledged that what it all boiled down to was the integrity of Ellen White's counsel.

For the first time in many, many months of discussion, the council's decision firmly established the future of a four-year medical curriculum at CME. Also, it authorized the construction of the White Memorial Hospital on the Los Angeles campus. Finally, CME administrators sensed that church officers at all levels overwhelmingly supported the success of the college.[14]

### The Women Get It Done

The "Women's Movement"[15] and the "Women's Committee on the Los Angeles Hospital,"[16] as they were known, wasted no time in beginning their fund-raising efforts. Before the historic Loma Linda meetings had adjourned, the ladies took pictures of a number of pioneering church brethren. They planned to sell the pictures for 50 cents each. Mrs. Haskell, chair of the group, later reported: "When the aged brethren heard that their photographs were to be sold for money, they at first objected, but when they learned that [they] would be used to build the Ellen G. White Memorial Hospital, they were glad to help."[17]

Although Ellen White died four months before the formal decision was made to build the hospital, W. C. White described visiting his mother on a rainy day near the end of her long, final illness. After talking with her for a little while, he told her that he had good news regarding the work at Loma Linda.[18]

"I then related that a good sister in the East [Mrs. Lida Scott] had offered to make a very liberal gift to the College of Medical Evangelists for the establishment of a students' home and hospital in Los Angeles.[19] Mother's lips quivered, and for a moment she shook with emotion. Then she said: 'I am glad you told me this. I have been in perplexity about Loma Linda, and this gives me courage and joy.'

"After a little further conversation I knelt down by her side and thanked the God of Israel for His manifold blessings, and prayed for a continuance of His mercies. Then Mother offered a very sweet prayer of about a dozen sentences, in which she expressed gratitude, confidence, love, and entire resignation."[20]

In later years this crucial time of decision was remembered with respect and humility. Reuben R. Figuhr, president of the General Conference in 1962, reviewed the early concerns over starting a hospital in Los Angeles:

"Some good brethren in the early years of our medical school felt that giving any part of the medical training in Los Angeles was a denial of the messages Sister White had brought to this people regarding the establishment of our sanitariums and schools. But she and our loyal, devoted leaders back there, whose memory we revere, did not think so. They were not establishing a sanitarium, but a hospital-clinic where there would be both an abundance of patients and a wide variety of different diseases. . . . At the very outset our leading brethren clearly saw this difference and moved forward accordingly."[21]

Then he quoted "good old Elder S. N. Haskell." We are told that "we *must provide* that which is essential, etc. A hospital in a large city where there are many poor is one of the essential things required by the laws of the land. [So] we are building it in Los Angeles, the nearest large city. Loma Linda is out in the country. The hospital will be built in the nearest place it can be built and meet the demands of the law."[22]

## CME's New Supervisor in Los Angeles

On November 25, 1915, the board took three important actions. First, they officially voted to ask Magan to join the faculty and to direct CME's educational program in Los Angeles. An astute educator, Magan had matured through hardship and sacrifice. The orator could always instill confidence in members of the church constituency. Because of a lack of funds, however, CME invited Magan to join its faculty under the condition that he raise his own salary ($23 per week).[23] Because of the physician's passionate loyalty to the denomination, he accepted the invitation despite the fact that he had medical school debts to pay and a successful practice in Nashville, which he had to give up, along with his educational responsibilities at Madison.

Second, the board chair was asked to "appoint a committee of five to furnish the sisters, who are planning to raise the funds with which to build a hospital and dispensary in Los Angeles, information regarding the need, object, etc., of the buildings in order that they may work intelligently in soliciting the funds, and to assist in the raising of the funds. Carried."[24]

Finally, Newton Evans introduced the possibility of conducting *both* of the clinical years of the medical course in Los Angeles instead of the last year only. A comprehensive discussion ensued. One or two members of the faculty were not convinced that it was the best thing to do—at least morally speaking. However, in light of potential accreditation, they "voted, that, after sufficient investigation, if it is found to be absolutely necessary to conduct the last two years in Los Angeles in order to secure the proper rating of the school, the Faculty be authorized to make this arrangement."[25]

### Another Report Card

In mid-December the Council on Medical Education inspected CME. At the time, no one was prepared for the devastating news that CME would retain its class C rating. The report, painful to read even today, provided a perspective of the accreditation concerns of the era. Understandably, this report caused major discouragement in Loma Linda. Nonetheless, administrators accepted it as a challenge and—thankful that the school had not been closed—mounted an appropriate response.

### Fund-raising for the Los Angeles Venture

On February 23, 1916, the board voted to appoint a committee of five to recommend a site for the hospital in Los Angeles, to present plans for the building, and to assist in the collection of funds for the project. They appointed L. M. Bowen, Newton G. Evans, Alfred Q. Shryock, S. S. Merrill, and John Burden to the committee.[26] On June 7, 1916, the board voted to approve the preliminary steps taken by the committee and secure the Michigan and Boyle Avenues property in Los Angeles, California, for $8,000.[27]

The *Review and Herald* publicized the fund-raising efforts. The Autumn Council of the North American Division Conference recommended that Mrs. Haskell should organize the movement with representative women from each union and local conference. The endeavor would be promoted by further articles in the *Review and Herald*, the union conference papers, by correspondence, and by personal solicitation.[29]

The women had other creative ideas. Some sisters in the church sewed and some made rugs and other articles. The Central California Conference appointed one woman from each congregation to coordinate the fund-raising enterprise. Because they lived in peach country some women picked peaches. One woman donated $3.50 as a result of her day's work. Even children caught the spirit. One little boy donated $1.25.[30]

## A Petition Letter From the CME Board to the Executive Committee of the North American Division (1916)

"Dear Brethren:

"Last fall it was arranged by the Division Conference Council held at Loma Linda, California, that a campaign should be inaugurated during the early part of 1916 to raise the sum of $61,000 for the erection of a hospital and dispensary for our medical school, the same to be erected in Los Angeles, California.

"Some of our sisters volunteered to undertake the raising of this sum of money. The North American Division Council authorized these women to undertake the raising of the above sum of money, offering to them their fullest cooperation. In order to assist them in their enterprise, Dr. P. T. Magan was recommended by the Board of the College of Medical Evangelists to enter the field and solicit large donations from our people in various sections of the country. Later the North American Division Committee advised the appointment of a Women's Committee in each Union and local conference to cooperate with the leaders of the Women's Movement in their endeavor to secure the above funds. . . . We feel that the Women's Movement should be helped by inaugurating a more active campaign in soliciting funds in various parts of the country."

The report, signed by Dr. Magan, contained a partial list of pledges already totaling $31,382.50. Elder and Mrs. John A. Burden gave $250, and medical students contributed $1,500. "Dr. Leroy Otis' little son pledged $40." A list of conditional pledges totaled $13,250 and included $1,000 from the St. Helena Sanitarium.[28]

As might be expected, the tireless Magan was at the forefront of the fundraising endeavors. On one of his first trips, he visited with his friend Paulson at the Hinsdale Sanitarium. While there he studied the testimonies from Ellen White about Loma Linda.

Experienced as he was, Magan still found this project utterly overwhelming. He wrote to Ellen White's son, W. C. White: "I cannot but feel that in Los Angeles I have undertaken the biggest contract in my life, and I know that without special help from God it will shipwreck me, for I am not big enough, nor man enough, and I do not have sense enough to put that thing through. It is beset with difficulties from every side."[31] He *knew* he could not survive without divine guidance.

After a day of difficult meetings at Loma Linda, he wrote in his diary: "In the evening I walked around the hill to my favorite seat and prayed for a long time. God strengthened me, and many things began to clear up in my mind. A sense of security in God came over me, and I knew that He is my Helper."[32]

### World War I Impacts CME

America entered World War I on April 6, 1917. Suddenly, the need to improve CME's accreditation status increased dramatically. By May 1 Congress had passed the Conscriptive Draft Act that made most CME faculty and students eligible for military service. It also affected premedical students across the nation who had hoped to be admitted into CME.

Meanwhile, bad press about the church's noncombatant religious conviction created prejudice in government circles. Magan clarified the church's position to Dr. Franklin H. Martin, a member of the advisory commission of the Department of Defense. Martin cordially requested that CME organize a base hospital that would be staffed entirely by Adventists and be made available for overseas service.

During an emergency meeting held in Loma Linda on July 3 and 4, 1917, Magan emphasized the need to discuss the denomination's relationship with the government. During this meeting the board voted unanimously to organize a base hospital in France. Even though the U.S. Army never accepted the offer, the action did change the opinion of some government officials toward Adventists.

In 1917 there were 99 schools of medicine in the United States: 71 class A schools, 16 class B schools, and 12 class C schools.[33] By August 1 of that year draft boards were conscripting medical students at an alarming rate, an action that impacted every school of medicine in America. The government had not made any provision for the continuation of medical education until August 31, 1917. Martin sent a telegram to CME: "A regulation providing for exemption of interns and medical students authorized by President."

### In the Valley of the Shadow

On August 30, 1917, the provost marshal general sent all state governors details of the supplemental regulations governing the execution of the selective service law. In it he identified all those who could join the Enlisted Reserve Corps, including sophomore, junior, and senior student physicians and interns, all of whom had to be students or graduates of "well-recognized medical schools." Or, if called by their local draft board, these same people could seek discharge from military service by enrolling in the Enlisted Reserve Corps of the Medical Department. The significant words "well-recognized medical schools," of course, challenged CME.

Because CME still maintained a class C rating with the American Medical Association, the national directive refused any of its students who sought exemption. The Army exempted schools whose graduates were accepted by 70 percent of the state examining boards, and not even 50 percent recognized CME. Evans and Magan considered the situation as the most serious crisis in the college's short history. If the school were to close under these circumstances, *it would never reopen.*

In an effort to win government recognition, Magan headed for Washington, D.C., to enlist the support of Army officers, physicians, and church leaders. He then arranged for Evans to bring Dr. George Hare, of Fresno, California, to a series of conferences in Chicago. President of the American Academy of Medicine, Hare strongly supported CME. On October 25, 1917, Magan, Evans, and Hare met with Colwell and Dr. George H. Simmons, general secretary of the American Medical Association. Decisions made there led to another visit to Washington, D.C., to the office of the surgeon general.

In the absence of the surgeon general, a General Noble and Colonel Love agreed to exempt all CME students from active military service. Thus, they could finish their medical education in Loma Linda, after which they would become medical officers. They based their agreement on the condition that the AMA would raise the rating of CME to a class B rating. The Army decided to return CME's drafted students, subject to the pending decision by the Council on Medical Education.[34]

Colwell promised to conduct an inspection within two weeks! In haste, Magan bombarded his administrative colleagues in Loma Linda and Los Angeles with mail and telegrams, urging them to prepare.

One directive went to Fred W. Drake, the superintendent of new construction in Los Angeles: "Spare no pains to push the work on the surgery building as fast as you can and a good deal faster. Get more men, get students to help, but get that building as near completed as you can. . . . Get that filthy crop of tin cans, rubber boots, cast-off clothing, and other elements of the abomination of desolation reaped with the sickle of the reaper and burned in your incinerator."

He advised Alfred Shryock, who was based at Loma Linda, to do his best, "to have everything at Loma Linda in apple-pie order." He wanted the hospital records, including autopsies, to be well organized, "so that nothing will be awry when he comes."

In one of his last letters to Bowen, the business manager at Loma Linda, Magan followed his instructions with a spiritual note: "The Lord has worked miracles for us thus far, and I do not want to see things fall down now through any fault of ours. You remember that expression in *The Story of Prophets and Kings*: 'God can work miracles for His people only as they act their part with untiring energy. He calls for men of devotion to His work, men of moral courage, with ardent love for souls, and with a zeal that never flags. Such workers will find no task too arduous, no prospect too hopeless; they will labor on, undaunted, until apparent defeat is turned into glorious victory.'"

This emergency prompted the board to further expand facilities in Los Angeles. On November 2, 1917, they voted to authorize the construction of two additional hospital buildings, administration and women's surgery, with the understanding that the school's rating would be raised to class B by the American Medical Association.[35]

### The Report Card: A Promotion!

On November 13, 1917, Colwell inspected CME thoroughly. As he said goodbye to Magan, he promised: "I will do my utmost to secure the raise in rating for you." The next day Colwell called to announce that a class B rating for CME could be assured.

A jubilant Magan immediately telegraphed the surgeon general, requesting the return of drafted CME medical students. He then wired each draftee: "Dr. Colwell has been here and has raised our rating to B Grade. Council on Medical Education will confirm telegram already gone to Surgeon General relative to you. . . . Letter follows. Leave matter in my hands, and keep confidential. Will rush matters as fast as possible. Notify the others."[36]

In his follow-up letter, Magan reported that he had spent the longest and hardest seven weeks of his life coping with the government. He tried to arrange for rights entitled to student physicians in good standing under the ruling of the surgeon general of the U.S. Army. Later, Magan told the CME constituency that the seven-week struggle and suspense he endured had turned out to be a walk of faith with God:

"There is something about the experience of having the burden of a great crisis rolled upon you when you are all alone [that] drives you very close to God. I was on my way to save the only medical school in all the world which bore the name of God. . . . From office to office and from one great man to another I went, but nowhere did I get a word of comfort. I remember one bitter cold day, with driving wind and snow, disheartened and not knowing what next to do, I left the office of the Surgeon General and sat down on the stone curbing supporting the iron fence around the White House. There I sat and prayed and there came into my mind some of the closing words in Solomon's great prayer at the dedication of the temple—'and let these my words . . . be nigh unto the Lord our God day and night, that He maintain the cause of His servant.'

"I remembered the prayers which so often fell from the lips of Ellen G. White, of John Burden, of many another soul who struggled to launch the school. I, too, had prayed and it came into my mind that prayers do not die when they leave our lips; they are 'nigh unto the Lord our God day and night.' I knew that prayers offered long ago were still doing duty before the great white throne, and I was comforted."[37]

On February 3, 1918, the Council on Medical Education unanimously confirmed Colwell's recommendation to upgrade CME's rating.[38] Now not only could former students return from military camps, but also the college could grow and, more importantly, fulfill its mission. Both faculty and General Conference officers considered the new class B rating to be temporary. CME *must* continue to improve its physical plant and the quality of its educational program in order to earn the necessary class A rating.

## The Ellen G. White Memorial Hospital

On Sunday, April 21, 1918, CME dedicated the 64-bed White Memorial Hospital in East Los Angeles.[39] It had been built from funds raised mostly by Ellen White's sisters in the church, under the leadership of Mrs. Haskell and with administrative support from Magan.[40]

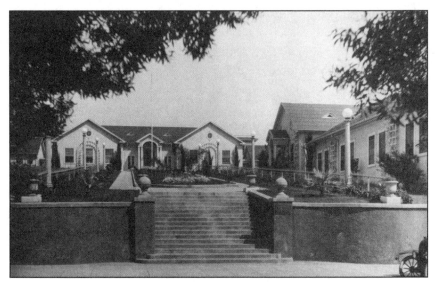

Often referred to as "The White," it was a cottage hospital built as a series of bungalows.

At the constituency meeting the next day, Newton Evans gave the presidential perspective on the recent upgrade of the school's rating with the AMA, and he outlined the challenges faced by the college and the consequences for its students. The favorable action by the Council on Medical Education of the American Medical Association enabled CME's draft-eligible students to continue their studies and those who had already been drafted to return to their schoolwork:

"On the first of June [1918] the fourth class of physicians was graduated from the school, but there have been impediments in various fields on account of the lack of such recognition on the part of the American Medical Association as has been necessary to secure legal recognition in many of the states of the Union. We have looked forward eagerly to the time when these conditions would be different and have prayed much that the time would come when the Lord could trust us with the favors which he held in store for the school. When it became evident on the first of October last year that the United States Government would not give us the recognition which was being given to the Medical Schools of the best reputation and which is necessary in order that the medical students may be released from the draft for military service, and allowed to continue their medical studies, active efforts were made by us to secure a change in the Government's attitude. The Lord signally blessed these efforts.

"With this recognition by the American Medical Association and the United States Government it became possible for our graduates to be legally licensed in most of the states of the Union, thus the conditions which threatened the very existence of the school were used of the Lord to bring a wonderful blessing. These events have impressed us with the sense of our absolute dependence on God's providences and the fact that our work is and must be entirely a work of faith. This should serve to make and keep us humble and to strengthen our trust."[41]

### The New Dispensary Enhances Clinical Experience

During the constituency meeting of April 22, 1918,[42] Magan reported the first seven weeks of progress at the Los Angeles Division's new dispensary. Before moving to the new facility, the dispensary had charged nothing. Then, in an effort to become self-supporting, the unit charged patients 10 cents per visit. Fortunately, charging the patients had no affect on attendance. Although some predicted that after moving into the new dispensary, patronage would drop, it didn't. In fact the patient load doubled from 50 patients a day to 100 a day.

Magan recognized the Adventist doctors who had stood by the institution "when we were in hard quarters." They had nobly given their services and donated any fee they collected for their work. These dedicated physicians had received no pay for any cases they had managed in the hospital. Based on their work and with the rapidly increasing work force, everyone had realized the importance of "every teacher and worker reaching the highest point of efficiency."

Everyone was pleased with the upgrade in CME's rating to the B class. On February 28, 1918, I. H. Evans, vice president of the General Conference, was caught up in the moment. Although he had been one of the most conservative in approving CME's expansion, he wrote to Magan: "I do hope to see the school within two years classified as 'A.' I believe we can make it if we are to operate a full-fledged school in class 'A' just as readily and just as successfully as in class 'B,' but I am very thankful that we have been lifted from class 'C.'"

The two years that I. H. Evans predicted and that everyone expected was not meant to be for a variety of reasons. World War I still raged, and the relationship of medical schools to the United States military became even more complex. In November 1918 a crisis developed that again threatened CME's survival.[43]

[1] *University Observer*, November 13, 1980; *The Medical Evangelist*, February 15, 1940, p. 4.

[2] A.V. Olsen, "George I. Butler Moves Into the Light," *Through Crisis to Victory* (Washington, D.C.: Review and Herald Publishing Association, 1966), pp. 90, 91.

[3] *The Medical Evangelist*, February 15, 1940, p. 4.

[4] Ellen G. White, MS 72-09, September 23, 1909; "The Relation of Loma Linda College to Worldly Medical Institutions," Paulson Collection, pp. 269-274.

[5] Ellen G. White, letter to John A. Burden, October 11, 1909, B 132-09.

[6] *The Medical Evangelist*, February 15, 1940, p. 4; November 1953, p. 9.

[7] *Ibid.*, February 15, 1940, p. 4.

[8] Loma Linda Fire Chief Francis Dinsmore documented this report on a wire recording at a Camp Cedar Falls retreat in 1949, Centennial Anniversary of CME/LLU—2005, Department of Archives and Special Collections, document file 3229.06.

[9] Department of Archives and Special Collections, Loma Linda University, document file 3229.06.

[10] Merlin L. Neff, "An 'Inspirator' for CME," *For God and CME*, p. 176.

[11] *The Medical Evangelist*, February 15, 1940, p. 4.

[12] Department of Archives and Special Collections, document file 3229.06.

[13] Keld J. Reynolds, Ph.D., "School Begins," *Outreach*, Loma Linda, California, 1968, p. 17.

[14] W. E. Macpherson, M.D., W. F. Norwood, Ph.D., "Far-reaching Decision on Locating CME on Two Campuses," *The Medical Evangelist*, November 1953, p. 9.

[15] CME board of trustees, minutes, May 16, 1916, p. 2.

[16] "Los Angeles Hospital," *Review and Herald*, December 16, 1915, pp. 8, 9.

[17] Mrs. S. N. Haskell, "The Veterans' Aid to the Hospital Fund," *Review and Herald*, April 27, 1916, p. 20; Albert F. Brown, M.D., "The White," *Diamond Memories*, p. 84.

[18] W. C. White, quoted by Arthur L. White, "The Last Mile," *The Elmshaven Years*, p. 429.

[19] CME board of trustees, minutes, June 15, 1915, p. 4.

[20] W. C. White, "The Los Angeles Hospital," *Review and Herald*, September 28, 1916; Arthur L. White, "The Last Mile," *The Elmshaven Years*, p. 429.

[21] Reuben R. Figuhr, "A Statement on Loma Linda University," *Review and Herald*, July 19, 1962, pp. 4-8.

[22] S. N. Haskell, quoted by Reuben R. Figuhr, "A Statement on Loma Linda University," *Review and Herald*, July 19, 1962, pp. 4-8.

[23] Newton G. Evans, M.D., letter to Edward A. Sutherland, M.D., December 23, 1915;

Percy T. Magan, M.D., letter to J. J. Ireland, January 27, 1917; "History," *Loma Linda University Magazine*, spring 1965, p. 38.

[24] CME board of trustees, minutes, November 25, 1915, p. 13.

[25] *Ibid.*

[26] *Ibid., February* 23, 1916, p. 4. On March 23, 1916, the board made the name of the proposed hospital official—Ellen G. White Memorial Hospital. Over time, the "Ellen G." part of the name was lost, thereby identifying less with the remarkable woman being honored.

[27] *Ibid.,* June 7, 1916, p. 2.

[28] *Ibid.*, May 16, 1916, pp. 2, 5-6.

[29] I. H. Evans and G. B. Thompson, "Los Angeles Hospital," *Review and Herald*, December 16, 1915, pp. 8, 9.

[30] "What the Women Are Doing," *Review and Herald*, September 28, 1916, p. 2.

[31] Percy T. Magan, letter to W. C. White, January 11, 1916.

[32] Percy T. Magan, diary, July 11, 1916.

[33] Alfred Q. Shryock, M.D., "The Story of Loma Linda," *The Medical Evangelist*, December 15, 1927, p. 2.

[34] Merlin L. Neff, "Through Deep Shadows of War," *For God and CME*, pp. 194-197.

[35] CME board of trustees, minutes, November 2, 1917, p. 458.

[36] Percy T. Magan, Telegram to F. M. Stump, et al., November 13, 1917.

[37] Percy T. Magan, "President's Report to the Constituency," minutes, January 28, 1940, pp. 12, 13.

[38] Percy T. Magan, letter to W. C. Knox, February 3, 1918.

[39] *College of Medical Evangelists Tenth Annual Announcement*, June 1918, p. 12.

[40] Albert F. Brown, M.D., "The White," *Diamond Memories*, p. 84.

[41] CME constituency meeting, minutes, April 22, 1918, pp. 1, 2.

[42] *Ibid.*, pp. 15-17, 19.

[43] Margaret Rossiter White, "The A Rating," *The Ministry*, October 1960, p. 33.

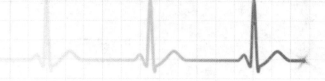

# Chapter 5

# Surviving Wartime Crises

### The Dismemberment of Medical School Faculties

By July 1918 a new crisis developed when the United States military began drafting schools of medicine faculty in key positions. This resulted in the disorganization of teaching staffs across the United States. After consulting with Colonel Horace D. Arnold, surgeon general of the War Department, Magan learned that every physician would have to join the Medical Reserve Corps or the Volunteer Service Corps of the Army.[1]

By enlisting in the Medical Enlisted Reserve Corps, CME's student physicians could continue their studies. They didn't even know they were in the Army, and their noncombatant status had been assured. In the fall of 1918, however, the government changed the original plan and notified all the deans of the nation's medical schools that their students must join the Students' Army Training Corps (SATC). Furthermore, they would be considered enlisted soldiers in the Army. Any school wanting to form its own unit had to apply to the government and had to have at least 100 men of college level.

### The Students' Army Training Corps (SATC)

Former president of CME and now the medical secretary of the General Conference, Ruble interviewed military officials in Washington, D.C., on behalf of CME. His investigation revealed that the War Department favored limiting recognition to schools that had a unit of the Students' Army Training Corps. Moreover, Colonel Arnold's office had told him that because CME did not have a sufficient number of students it would probably receive no further consideration. Ruble even learned that there likely would be only one surviving school of medicine in California and that the University of California had already received that distinction.

This development could very easily close CME. In crisis mode once again, the board convened on September 20, 1918, and voted unanimously to apply for a unit of the Students' Army Training Corps. To achieve the numbers required, they would create affiliations with the University of Redlands and Occidental College in Los Angeles. Because regulations also covered premedical students, they would also start a premedical department for up to 25 students from Pacific Union College (Angwin, California). Then they would be available to join Loma Linda's proposed SATC.[2]

Church leaders on the West Coast could see only one way to save the school of medicine and to prevent disrupting the studies of their medical and premedical students—joining the SATC. The presidents of Walla Walla College (Walla Walla, Washington) and Union College (Lincoln, Nebraska) monitored developments with increasing interest. Working together to make up the numbers seemed to be the only solution for everyone.

### To Join or Not to Join

The subject of combatant *versus* noncombatant further compounded the problem. To discuss the enormous problem, Ruble called together a special meeting of church leaders in Washington, D.C., on Sabbath, September 14. His report to Magan forecast the storm of opposition to come. The possibility that students at Seventh-day Adventist colleges could lose their noncombatant status aroused grave concern.

On the other hand, Ruble and his colleagues at CME believed that medical service in the Army Reserve equaled being a noncombatant. Assurances from government officials in California supported their position. Could CME meet government requirements to form an SATC unit in order to avoid closing the school? This became a vital concern for Magan and Evans.

They moved quickly to determine whether the University of Redlands and Occidental College would join their cause. They also sought advice and support from Dr. Ray Lyman Wilbur, president of Stanford University and regional director of the SATC program. Wilbur immediately wired Washington and recommended acceptance of the proposed Loma Linda unit. The administrators of CME, Walla Walla College, Pacific Union College, and Union College waited for a reply to Wilbur's letter.

Then began a rush of telegraph activity, crisscrossing the country. The Education Department of the General Conference stepped in, sending a telegram and a long letter expressing strong disapproval of the plan: "Committee has not authorized any of these steps and fear you are compromising the denomination."

Clearly, denominational leaders felt that anyone joining an SATC unit would forfeit his noncombatant status. Evans quickly wired church leaders suggesting that they had *not* studied Magan's explanation. In response, a night letter from Daniells and F. W. Howell illustrated the dynamics of the crisis:

"Advice obtained from military authorities revealed that those joining the Medical Reserve of SATC become combatants, forfeiting noncombatant standing, hence General Conference Committee in full session, Ruble present, decided it cannot authorize premedical work at Loma Linda nor advise formation [of] SATC in denominational institutions."[3]

J. H. Christian, president of the CME Board of Trustees, Evans, Magan, and others responded with yet another night letter on September 29: "Your wire has caused us deep perplexity. Board met. With all courtesy believe you absolutely misunderstand situation in which you place us. . . . Following your counsel school must close immediately. We have information that once closed it will never be permitted to reopen. Officials with whom we have counseled have assured us that noncombatant status will not be compromised by training corps in medical school. We have acted in good faith."

To complicate matters still further, Magan received a telegram on October 2 from Wilbur. According to officials in Washington, D.C., he said, the War Department had received no application for an SATC unit at Loma Linda. In any case, no additional units were going to be established.

To enlist support for Loma Linda's noncombatant position, Magan wired Adjutant General James J. Borree, an attorney in Sacramento. He requested a positive statement regarding those with conscientious scruples being called to bear arms. He reminded General Borree that President Woodrow Wilson had designated the Medical Corps as a *noncombatant* service. Borree's reply on October 5 was not helpful: "Opinion of this office medical student who enters army training corps forfeits right to noncombatant service. Signed, Borree."

## Can We Keep CME Open?

How would CME respond? Administrators firmly believed that CME had been established under divine guidance and, with faith, prayer, and sacrifice developed for the training of medical missionaries. Even under these difficult circumstances, they would not give up. They called an emergency meeting in Oakland from October 7 to 11, 1918, to discuss the issues.

Following Wilbur's recommendation, they decided to send Magan to Washington, D.C., to petition the War Department. "We want to establish a noncombatant SATC in Loma Linda." Magan planned to join Dr. George Thomason, who was already in the nation's capital. Together they would meet with Major General E. H. Crowder, provost marshal, the adjutant general of the Army. If necessary, they would attempt to reach President Wilson himself.

At this critical time Magan succumbed to the influenza pandemic that was sweeping the world (1918-1919).[4] He gave up his plans to travel east. Although burdened with heavy responsibilities, including the startup of the wartime nursing school in Loma Linda, Evans quickly decided to go in Magan's place. With supporting documents, he entrained for Washington, D.C., where he met Thomason on October 29. The CME physicians found the nation's capital almost paralyzed by the influenza epidemic.

Back on the West Coast students were becoming restless. Tensions mounted while they waited for Evans' reports. As one group of students after another were taken for physical examinations, church members fasted and prayed. A stream of telegrams reported step-by-step progress to the college presidents. Amid the ebb and flow of opinions, emotions also rose and fell by the hour. One wire stated that CME's request would be considered. Another asserted that a noncombatant corps was out of the question. A final telegram declared that all government officials had insisted that training corps students were combatants. Church officials, however, would not consent to opening a training corps.

Although not fully recovered from his bout with influenza, Magan would not give up. He called a special board meeting where he and Christian drafted a night letter to Evans. They feared that if circumstances forced students to attend other schools in order to join the SATC, they would feel that the denomination had deserted them after they had faithfully stood by.

The doctors expressed their opinion that "to close the college [was a] bigger violation of the Testimonies [from Ellen G. White] than to have [the] corps." Further, they urged Evans to go the limit and petition President Wilson to allow a special corps at Loma Linda.

## A Miraculous End to the Crisis

The negotiations with the government were becoming more and more complicated and unsolvable. Then World War I ended. Students on their way to military service suddenly returned home. The armistice of November 11, 1918, indeed, saved the College of Medical Evangelists. Magan believed that God's hand was evidenced in the timeliness of the armistice in what he called, "the sudden, spectacular and miraculous close of the war."[5]

Evans agreed: "Again we felt that the hand of Providence had intervened. . . . In our experience in the school we have come to expect trials and difficulties and to believe that these are permitted to help us to continue to realize our absolute dependence upon God and His upholding and protecting care."[6]

Once again CME had survived—it would live to fight even more battles against its very existence.

## Picking Up the Postwar Pieces

By 1919 CME was operating the largest and by far the best-equipped dispensary in the city of Los Angeles. According to Magan, it scheduled more than 18,000 patient visits in 1918, about one third more than the oldest dispensary in town. Beyond the statistics, he cherished the general feeling of confidence and brotherly love expressed toward the White Memorial Hospital by the world church: "I don't know that I have ever spent a year of my life in any institution when I have had greater reason to believe that our General [Conference] Brethren in Washington [D.C.] and our local men were really heart and soul with us, and doing all they could do to help us and more than we dreamed they could or would do. . . . I feel this is a matter which ought to give all of us a great deal of thankfulness—to our God and to our brethren."[7]

World War I had definitely impacted CME's enrollment. Magan felt strongly that enrollment needed to increase in order to keep the school open.

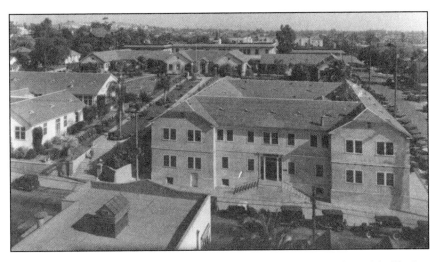

The enlarged outpatient dispensary on the right is surrounded by the "cottage hospital," named the Ellen G. White Memorial Hospital.

A letter from the government stated that small schools of medicine would be joined to large schools in an effort to provide more physicians to the military. Magan used this information to emphasize the need for CME to recruit more church members. "I cannot believe the Lord wrought the wonderful providence that He did, then to have the school closed up because we do not have a large attendance," he said.

The old class C rating had turned many potential students away from CME. Now that CME had a higher rating, Magan proposed that the church make a "tremendous effort" to recruit SDA medical students from worldly schools. Sabbath difficulties not only existed there, but they probably would increase due to the military requirement of reducing the curriculum from four years to three.[8]

The new rating was a cause for celebration and an opportunity to recruit more students. General Conference President Daniells called for gratitude and praise:

"We do not indulge very much in praise of each other or throwing bouquets to persons, but I feared perhaps I did not give enough glory to God, because it does seem to me, brethren, that the Lord has taken hold and wrought changes here Himself in this situation. I know plenty of men who could not believe that this rating would be raised, and they were sincere men and thoughtful men—men of good judgment in things—preachers, and doctors who put it right down hard and flat to me with a thump on the table that we would never get this thing raised. We were down in a hole and would never get out of it. They believed it and were sincere, and they didn't wish the institution ill either. A great many of us had grave fears and anxiety about it. The thing seemed stupendous. It seemed impossible when you looked at it from one standpoint. But it swung around and we are there. Now away back behind all the scenes of perplexity and strife, many humble people were on their knees praying, and I suppose there is just as much credit due them as to those who went down to Washington and met the medical men. It is the people who get down and fight these battles out in the dark and get victory through faith and prayer. I guess we are all in it. It's the people who gave their money. But to God belongs the glory and the power for working this change and putting it where it is."[9]

Observers attributed much of the credit for changing the rating to Magan and Hare and their professional associations with influential people in the area of medical education. Not seeking credit for himself, Magan acknowledged God's intervention and the good faith of the students.

"I do not think I shall ever forget as long as I live one day in Washington and one in Chicago, when men, big men medically, big men of the world who had for years told us, 'You never can succeed, you cannot put that thing over,' when these men kindly and quietly and seemingly with deep feeling in their hearts, told us, 'We have come to believe that your cause is right and we are going to help you.' I believe, brethren, with all my heart that the angels of God heard prayers uttered all over the land and turned those men's hearts in our time of need. I will never to my dying day believe that it was anything else but the mighty power of God that turned these men's hearts. I think you have heard me tell how one of those men had been labored with for hours—how that man kindly, almost tenderly turned toward Doctor Hare and myself and gave us his hand and said, 'I will do everything in my power to help you.' I believe that was the power of the almighty God....

"It has taken a great deal of faith on [the part of the students] to stay in school. I will never forget the afternoon I received the wire saying that the students had gotten together and said they would stick by the school even though it meant the trenches—instead of going to a worldly school. I thought then God was going to honor the faith of these poor lads. They turned their backs on all the favors other schools could give as far as military exemption was concerned. When I got that wire I knew in my soul that God would not desert us but would honor those young men and see them through."[10]

Concluding his part in this "review-and-praise" meeting, Magan offered an illustration:

"Dr. Ralph Smith accepted a commission and has gone as a medical officer of the Reserve Corps. The first thing he was asked to attend classes on Sabbath. . . . He took his stand that he would have to tell the officer he could not do it. He stood true on that. Then they put the examinations on the Sabbath. He sent back word again, 'I cannot do it. I have got to be true to my God.' I believe if our boys would take their stand strongly for God in the smaller experiences that come to them in their early days in the military service, when it comes to the big struggles that God is going to see them through. . . . I believe that God has saved the school that these men might be lights in the world."[11]

## Looking Ahead in 1919

CME's new hospital facilities were so well received that student physicians from outside schools sought admission. In 1919 CME admitted three junior and one senior transfer students from class A schools of medicine.[12] By July 1919 the White Memorial Hospital had enlarged to 75 beds,[13] and by 1922 to 120 beds.[14]

---

[1]Except where otherwise noted, most of the following scenario is condensed from Margaret Rossiter White, "The A Rating," *The Ministry*, October 1960, pp. 33-37.

[2]CME board of trustees, minutes, September 20, 1918, p. 1.

[3]A. G. Daniells and F. W. Howell, night letter to Newton G. Evans, M.D., September 28, 1918.

[4]Just as World War I was ending, the influenza pandemic of 1918-1919 killed more people than had died in the war itself. Somewhere between 20 and 40 million people perished in the most devastating epidemic in recorded world history.

[5]Margaret Rossiter White, loc. cit.

[6]CME constituency meeting, minutes, March 26, 1919, p. 2.

[7]CME board of trustees, minutes, March 26, 1919, p. 6.

[8]*Ibid.*, p. 19.

[9] *Ibid.*, p. 24.
[10] *Ibid.*, p. 26.
[11] *Ibid.*, p. 27.
[12] *The Medical Evangelist*, June 1919, p. 10.
[13] *College of Medical Evangelists Eleventh Annual Announcement*, July 1919, p. 20.
[14] *College of Medical Evangelists Fourteenth Annual Announcement*, August 1922, p. 19.

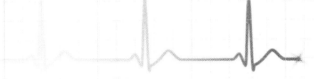

Chapter 6:

# A Tradition of Academic Hospitality

On April 18, 1920, the CME board learned that the University of Southern California (USC) would close its medical department at the end of the year "due to financial difficulties."[1] As a result, 15 of its medical students applied to CME, requesting to finish their medical education at the college. The majority of these students would enter their senior year. After careful consideration, the board "voted, to favor accepting as many of these applicants as shall be thought advisable by the executive officers of the school, with the understanding that on the completion of their medical course, the school from which they come will issue the degrees."[2]

### Closure of University of Southern California's School of Medicine

By June 1920, following the closing of the University of Southern California's school of medicine, CME became the fifth school of medicine in Southern California—and the only accredited one.[3] *This* was the school that Dr. John Harvey Kellogg once categorically declared to be "an enterprise that has no future!"[4] It also gained access to the vast patient resources of the recently enlarged 1,400-bed Los Angeles County Hospital. In fact, many of the volunteers who had been faculty at the University of Southern California now happily joined CME's faculty.[5]

Early in 1921 Newton Evans reported the arrangement to the constituency: "It will be well to explain briefly the occasion for the presence of the special medical students from the University of Southern California mentioned above. Some time last Spring the Board of Trustees of the University of

Southern California suddenly announced that the Medical Department at that school would be discontinued at the end of the school year 1919-[19]20. This left a large number of their students in a very difficult situation for various reasons and as a result of this situation numbers of their students as well as the teachers in the Medical School, earnestly begged us to make plans to accommodate at least their senior and junior classes. A great deal of time and study were given this problem, by our Board and Faculty, and it was finally decided to accept all of such senior and junior students as it seemed necessary to take on account of the difficulty of their finding other schools in which to finish their work. There were about twenty such senior students and fifteen juniors. It was arranged that for the most part their class work and clinics should be conducted in separate classes from our own medical students and practically all of the old medical teachers in the University of Southern California kindly consented to help in the task of carrying these two classes through until the time of graduation. These plans have been carried out and the work seems to be going along smoothly and satisfactorily. Classrooms for these students are provided in the Los Angeles County Hospital."[6]

## Loma Linda's Spiritual "Additive"

During this same time period the Loma Linda Sanitarium was thriving. Dr. H. W. Vollmer, the medical superintendent at the sanitarium, spoke to the constituency about the institution's spiritual life: "At present there are about 100 patients in the sanitarium and hospital. Nearly all the rooms in the main building are occupied. There is every indication, in spite of the financial depression, that we shall have a good patronage this winter. We are getting a very nice class of patients. A large number are very much interested in Bible study. It is real encouraging to see the interest they are taking in the religious services of the institution, and we feel confident that seed is being sown which in due time will reap a harvest of souls. Our guests appreciate the religious atmosphere of the institution and interest taken in their spiritual welfare."[7]

At the constituency meeting the following year (March 22, 1922), Magan described the spiritual atmosphere at the White Memorial Hospital and its impact on some of the USC students:

"As far as the religious work in the hospital is concerned, there are some things which I think will be of quite a little interest. We have had quite a deep religious experience among some of our nurses, and recently two of our nurses were converted and baptized.

"You will all remember with what misgivings we took hold of the matter of trying to train and help the students of the Southern California Medical College. There was considerable feeling that they might lead us astray and be a detriment to the school. Of course you realize most of their work was carried on at the Los Angeles County Hospital. One of those classes passed on and was graduated by the University last spring. Sixteen of their students remain with us in what came to us in a Junior class and will finish this year. We have all noticed, and noticed with a great deal of happiness and joy, the influence which our teachers and school [have] had over them.

"I think Doctor Coyne and Doctor Keller will bear me out that they do not make us a bit of trouble, and they mingle among us much the same as our own folks, eat at our cafeteria, and generally behave themselves in a most quiet and Christian manner.

"Two things of special interest have occurred. One of those students became converted, was baptized and joined our church, and I would like the privilege of reading a few lines which I received from this student, who is now a physician, graduated last spring, Dr. Judith Ahlem. She is taking an internship in the Alameda County Hospital.[8]

" 'I have missed you people of the White Memorial so much. Although I never seem to be able to live up to the principles of our church, yet I am glad that I can try—and I am glad that the dear Lord has answered so many of my prayers, because it makes me feel that my life may not be in vain after all. It has been my joyful privilege to speak a few words of the precious Truth to a few of my patients here. I wish you could have seen the smile of happiness that passed over the face of a repentant criminal (a mere lad of 18 years) when he was told that his sins could be forgiven. (At first he didn't really think it possible.) He asked to be told more of the word of God, said he had learned a hard lesson, and that he would begin life anew. That was all a week ago. He has now become desperately ill—perhaps but a few hours left to him now. I have spoken a few words to his mother now. She is surprised that there is a "Christian doctor." (I wish she knew a better one.)

" 'I shall always be grateful to you and those others who made it possible for us (USC) to come to your school. I also want you to remember that the

life of at least me was thereby much changed for good. That may not be saying much perhaps, just now, but it will mean more in the future.

"'(Signed) Judith Ahlem.'"[9]

"That letter touched me very much. The girl had a deep religious experience and has gone forth on a bright faith with this truth in her heart, into
the world." ·

## From USC to CME: A Thank-you Note

Magan was eager to share "one more little thing" about the USC transfer students. A
committee of the 16 remaining students "waited on him" with a letter:

Dear Doctor Magan:

As a class we have not been unmindful of the kindness which your Board of Trustees
has extended to us these last two years in assuming our burdens and making it possible for us to continue our medical course. Nor shall we forget the share which you personally have had in the situation, and the interest you have shown in us. It is because
this service has been given so unstintingly and in such a spirit of brotherly love that we
feel powerless to repay.

You may be sure of our lasting gratitude, and to that we wish to add the enclosed contribution toward the sum you are seeking to obtain for the medical school. Our regret is
that we are unable to make this commensurate with the deep appreciation we feel.

With most heart good will and best wishes from

The USC Contingent

In the envelope were checks and currency amounting to five dollars from every member
of that division. Each one chipped in the same amount [that] all of our students had
been trying to raise from their own ranks.[10]

## Oral Roberts University

Many years later, in 1989, history repeated itself when the school of medicine accepted student physicians from the Oral Roberts University School

of Medicine (Tulsa, Oklahoma). The sudden closure left many students stranded. Loma Linda University accepted student physicians from the first– , second–, and third–year classes. The Association of American Medical Colleges appreciated the decision and the event generated favorable coverage by the news media.[11]

Dr. Lyn Behrens, then dean of the school of medicine, provided perspective: "Loma Linda University School of Medicine was requested by the Liaison Council on Medical Education and Oral Roberts University School of Medicine to assist with the placement of transfer students. We were approached because of our distinctive Christian philosophy and because we share some of the same Christian values."[12]

The Oral Roberts University students were interested in Loma Linda University's overt Christian orientation. A special committee[13] interviewed 85 students during a one-day visit to Oklahoma. Although the school of medicine felt committed to students from California, the committee told other students that if they chose to come to Loma Linda and had the academic credentials, they too would be accepted.

Subsequently, the school offered acceptances to 21 freshmen, 14 sophomores, and 14 juniors. Names of students accepted were telephoned to Oklahoma on Wednesday evening, September 20, 1989. The list was posted at 6:30 a.m. the next morning. Within an hour some of the student physicians were on their way to Loma Linda. At the other end, CME student physicians offered to share living quarters with the new students while more permanent housing was located.[14]

Once again, Loma Linda extended "academic hospitality."

## A Curriculum Change

On March 23, 1922, the board's committee on plans and recommendations suggested that the medical college faculty inaugurate, as early as possible, the requirement of an intern year for completion of the medical course. Students then would receive a certificate of completion at the end of four years, but not their medical degree until completion of the fifth year.[15]

In 1927 the board voted to adopt a form of certificate to be issued to medical students upon the completion of their four years of study, the same to be signed by the dean and the president.[16]

This five-year arrangement lasted for the next 31 years until 1953 when student physicians started receiving their degrees after completing four years of medical school. In adjusting for the new arrangements, CME graduated two classes that year: the classes of 1953 -A and B.

## The Report Card Again, With Honors

The "March of CME" continued. After 12 years of effort by Loma Linda administrators and AMA councilmen, God blessed the hard work, financial sacrifices, and prayers of many. On November 14, 1922, the AMA Council on Medical Education awarded the College of Medical Evangelists the long-sought-after class A rating. CME then became the only class A medical school in Southern California. The new designation vindicated institutional leaders in their relentless pursuit of excellence in the face of ongoing setbacks, opposition, and discouragement.

At this time, Colwell, who was still serving as the secretary to the Council on Medical Education and Hospitals, confided to Magan:

"I never thought you people would succeed. I said so to you and to everyone else. But today my unbelief bows to the triumph of your faith, and no one is more glad and happy that you have succeeded than I am. When I was first shown the block upon which your plant is now located, it was covered with thistles and cockleburs, and one or two dilapidated-looking animals were grazing there. The doctor who was with me remarked: 'Someday we shall have a great medical institution here.' I thought to myself: I greatly fear they will never realize their ambition in this. But today I saw that same block entirely transformed, covered with buildings admirably adapted to their purposes, and a veritable hive of medical teaching activities."[17]

---

### CME's Promotion to Class A Rating[18]

Dear Dr. Magan:

After watching the efforts you have been making to develop your medical school during the past several years, it is my most pleasing duty to inform you that at its business meeting on November 14th, the Council on Medical Education and Hospitals voted that the College of Medical Evangelists be granted a class A rating.

Considering the manner in which improvements in the past have been made, the Council voted this higher rating fully confident that the places which are still comparatively weak will be strengthened, and that the institution will continue to improve.

You are undoubtedly already fully familiar with the fact that improvements can be made with great advantage in the following particulars: (a) further enlargement and improvement of the medical library at Los Angeles, (b) the making of adequate provision whereby medical research can be carried on, and (c) that the best methods of clinical instruction be installed for seniors at the bed-side of patients in the hospital, in the establishing of clinical clerkships, etc.

With sincere congratulations for the favorable action by the Council and with best wishes for the further development of your medical school, I am

Very truly yours,
N. P. Colwell, Secretary
Council on Medical Education and Hospitals[19]

Dr. Magan replied:

"To say that your letter brought happiness to the hearts of the little group of men who have struggled to make this Medical School worthy of the honor you have bestowed upon us, is to state our feelings very mildly indeed. I think I can truthfully say that this was the most blessed piece of information which has come to us since we commenced our long, long struggle."[20]

Later, Colwell wrote another letter that demonstrated the impact that CME and its mission had made on his life:

"I feel ashamed of myself sitting here rating you people, which is a little bit of a job, while you are doing the really big things of the world. You have done wonders in your school, and I am proud of you; and while you have not converted me to the seventh-day Sabbath as yet, you have converted me on practically everything else about your medical work."[21]

The board requested that the president of the faculty express the institution's appreciation to the Council on Medical Education and Hospitals. The awarding of a class A rating prompted them to disseminate the good news "as far as considered advisable."[22]

## A Climate Change for CME

Newton Evans described some of the circumstances relating to Colwell's latest visit. Magan had arranged for a luncheon attended by a number of CME's leading teachers and some of the medical friends in Los Angeles. A number of the guests spoke very appreciatively of the work of the school of medicine—much to the satisfaction of CME's leaders.

"All of our medical friends, as well as Colwell, who spoke, emphasized in their remarks the fact that they recognized that the College of Medical Evangelists is a school which is conducted for an entirely different purpose—namely, a medical missionary purpose, from the other schools of the country and that the work of the school is carried on in a different way, and that we have in our school an entirely different class of students than those attending the ordinary medical school.

"Colwell spoke with great feeling and sincerity. In all of his dealings with CME, he had recognized the studied effort of its leaders to be absolutely fair and honest in all of their relations with him. He deeply appreciated the spirit and principles he had found in this place."[23]

## Class A Benefits

The class A rating by the American Medical Association influenced licensing authorities throughout the United States. The A grade also opened doors for CME graduates to be tested by the National Board of Medical Examiners, whose certificates were recognized by various departments of the United States government and carried considerable weight in foreign countries.[24] In fact, because of the upgrade, medical missionary graduates could now take board examinations in many countries that previously had been closed to them.[25]

After the award of the A rating, the National Board of Medical Examiners, a comparatively new organization in the United States, recognized CME. It even held its examinations for the southwestern United States at the White Memorial Hospital. In due course Magan received a letter from the board management complimenting CME on the splendid test results achieved by its students. "They wrote an almost brotherly letter, I think one of the kindest and most friendly letters I have ever received from a Board of that kind in my life." Magan continued his historical perspective and outlined the practical consequences:

"Now you will bear in mind that we were not permitted to send our graduates and students against this examination at all until we received our "A" rating. It is only graduates or students of "A" grade schools who are allowed to take this examination. But once they have taken that and passed it successfully there are approximately thirty-three states in the Union in which they can practice without further examination or difficulty. . . . In all probability it will only be a short time until every state in the Union will recognize the examination of the National Board of Medical examiners."[26]

One of the school's pioneering faculty members, Alfred Shryock, truly understood the accreditation accomplishment and what it meant: "This [A rating] should be a cause for gratitude on our part and also should cause us to be very humble, for it was the Lord who did this for us and it indicates to us that we should be very careful to follow the Lord's leading here at Loma Linda so that He can accomplish His purposes through this institution. He has pointed out that a great work is to be accomplished by the graduates

### Proposal for CME's New Surgical Hospital in Loma Linda (Constituency Meeting, February 28, 1923)

1. It would free the original hospital to be used as a chapel, classrooms, and a much-needed men's residence hall.

2. It would free the cottages on the hill for sanitarium patient use, including a maternity unit. Some of the cottages had been housing male students.

3. It would concentrate all of the patient care activities of the institution on the hill.

4. Housing the male students together in the original hospital for the first time would provide for their support and supervision.

5. It would separate patient care activities from the sometimes-noisy student activities and playgrounds on the lower campus.

6. It would concentrate all of CME's educational activities in the three buildings on campus.[30]

of this institution and we need to walk softly before Him so that His purposes for us and for this school shall not be defeated."

The new rating had a ripple effect. On the day the Boyle Avenue Dispensary had opened, the institution happily served 23 patients. In 1922, the year of the rating upgrade, the dispensary served 60,000 patients.[27]

## A New Hospital on the Hill Beautiful

On March 23, 1922, Newton Evans suggested to the board that CME remodel the original Loma Linda Hospital on the lower campus to be used as college classrooms and a men's dormitory. These adjustments would follow as soon as a new hospital was erected on the hill. The board voted "to look with favor on some such plans."[28] Three months later, Evans reiterated his desire to see the school and sanitarium use the original hospital for dormitory and classroom space. Also, he suggested using the cottages on the hill for hospital purposes.[29]

Even before Evans' presentation of the proposal for a new hospital in Loma Linda, J. M. Cartwright had been asked to draw up building plans. His design called for a two-story structure. The basement would house treatment rooms,

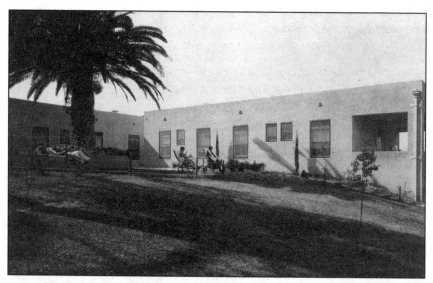

CME built the first section of Loma Linda's second "Hospital on the Hill" in 1924. This is the earliest-known photo of what is now the west end of Nichol Hall, showing an open-air porch.

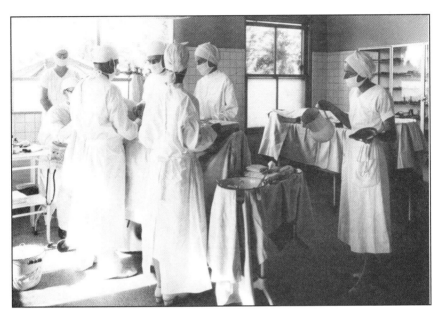

Surgery in progress at the second Loma Linda Hospital.

medical offices, operating rooms, guest rooms, and wards for surgical patients. Cartwright suggested that the new hospital be located in the orange grove on the ridge of the hill, south of the sanitarium. Upon completing his plans, he was to submit estimates for the cost of construction.

Cartwright projected the total investment for building the new hospital, remodeling the existing facilities, and purchasing some new equipment at $60,000.

Nonetheless, F. E. Corson, the comptroller, said that the first floor of the new unit (now the west end of Nichol Hall) would contain medical and dental offices, hydrotherapy and X-ray facilities, and examination rooms. This move would vacate 32 of the best rooms on the first and second floors of the sanitarium. The second floor of the new hospital would provide space for operating rooms and accommodations for about 20 inpatients.

Inadequate funds notwithstanding, the board of trustees voted to implement the action of the March 1, 1923, constituency meeting. As usual, the plans were fully carried out. Completed on August 24, 1924, the new hospital anchored the west end of what became the Loma Linda Sanitarium and Hospital in 1929.

## The Loma Linda Bowl

On February 7, 1924, the board considered constructing an outdoor amphitheater. Indeed, some work had already been done on the grounds of the amphitheater. Later, it became known as "The Loma Linda Bowl."[31] The last graduation ceremony was conducted in the Bowl on June 11, 1950. Eight years later, the board voted to demolish this hilltop landmark.[32]

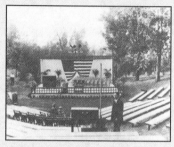

The outdoor amphitheater before the March 1935 remodel which added an acoustic shell and orchestra pit. Afterward it was referred to as the Loma Linda Bowl.

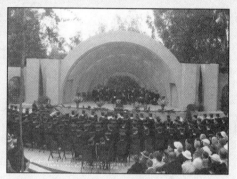

The 1935 graduation ceremony for the College of Medical Evangelists held in the Loma Linda Bowl.

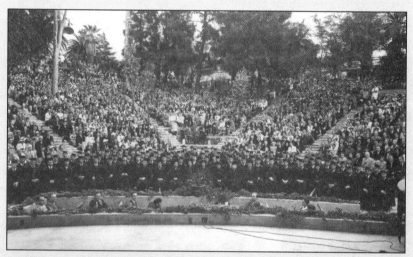

In 1938 the board approved enlarging the Loma Linda Bowl by moving fire hydrants, building new walkways, and increasing the seating capacity by 500 to 1,000.[33]

## Loma Linda Ideals Visualized

While working as an engineer in a top-secret government job, Glenn Rasmussen designed and built a piece of equipment for the War Department (now the Department of Defense). Later, he learned that his invention was part of the triggering mechanism for the atomic bomb. He felt so depressed that he told his wife that he wanted to spend the rest of his life saving people's lives. He wanted to become a physician.

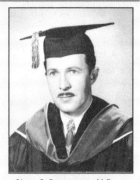

Glenn S. Rasmussen, M.D.

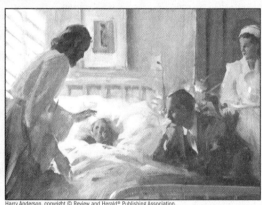

Harry Anderson, copyright © Review and Herald® Publishing Association.

The first draft of "The Consultation." As president of the CME class of 1950, Rasmussen is credited with commissioning this watercolor painting by Harry Anderson. He rejected this version, however, saying that he wanted to depict Christ working through the physician.

Now hanging in the offices of the Loma Linda University School of Medicine Administration, the final form of "The Consultation" met Rasmussen's requirements. Christ stands between the physician and the patient, linking the two together.

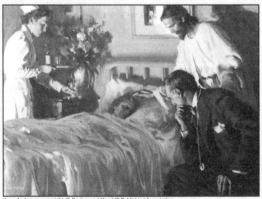

Harry Anderson, copyright © Review and Herald® Publishing Association.

[1] Helen Eastman Martin, M.D., *The History of the Los Angeles County Hospital (1878-1968)* (Los Angeles, California: University of Southern California Press, 1979), p. 91.

[2] CME board of trustees, minutes, April 18, 1920, pp. 1, 2.

[3] Merlin L. Neff, "The End of the Long, Long Battle," *For God and CME,* p. 217; Richard Utt, "If They Held Together, They Would Continue Strong," *From Vision to Reality, 1905-1980* (Loma Linda, California: Loma Linda University Press, 1980), p. 154; "They Have Gone and Done What I Told Them Not To," *The Vision Bold* (Washington, D.C.: Review and Herald Publishing Association, 1977), p. 198; Walter E. Macpherson, M.D., "The County," *Diamond Memories*, p. 77.

[4] John Harvey Kellogg, M.D., February 9, 1916, letter to Percy T. Magan, M.D.

[5] *College of Medical Evangelists Eleventh Annual Announcement*, July 1919, p. 20.

[6] CME constituency meeting, minutes, January 30, 1921, p. 3. In 1921 CME graduated 33 medical students from the University of Southern California.

[7] *Ibid.*, p. 6.

[8] *Ibid.*, March 22, 1922, p. 8.

[9] *Ibid.*, pp. 8, 9.

[10] *Ibid.*, p. 9

[11] *Ibid.*, October 4, 1989, p. 4; September 21, 1989, p. 2; LLUMC board of trustees, minutes, September 20, 1989, p. 1.

[12] B. Lyn Behrens, M.B., B.S., "Medicine Accepts Nearly 50 Oral Roberts' Students," *Scope*, October-December 1989, p. 20.

[13] The committee for the Oral Roberts acceptances: Dr. Behrens, John G. Kerbs, Ed.D., associate dean for admissions; William M. Hooker, Ph.D., associate dean for student affairs; and W. Barton Rippon, Ph.D., dean of the Graduate School.

[14] Behrens, p. 20.

[15] CME board of trustees, minutes, March 23, 1922, p. 2.

[16] *Ibid.*, May 5, 1927, pp. 5, 6.

[17] Nathan P. Colwell, M.D., *The Medical Evangelist*, May-June 1923, p. 4.

[18] On November 23, 1922, the CME board voted to incorporate into the minutes the official letter from Dr. Colwell. A copy of Colwell's letter is found on page 62 of *From Vision to Reality*.

[19] CME board of trustees, minutes, November 23, 1922, p. 3.

[20] Percy T. Magan, *From Vision to Reality*, p. 63.

[21] Nathan P. Colwell, M.D., *The Medical Evangelist*, May-June 1923, p. 4.

[22] CME board of trustees, minutes, November 23, 1922, p. 3.

[23] CME constituency meeting, minutes, February 28, 1923, p. 4.

[24] *Ibid.*

[25] Terrie Dopp, "Make It All You Possibly Can," *Scope*, October-December 1980, p. 21.

[26] CME constituency meeting, minutes, March 24, 1924, p. 24.

[27] *The Medical Evangelist*, May-June 1923, p. 4.

[28] CME board of trustees, minutes, March 23, 1922, pp. 4, 5.

[29] *Ibid.*, June 15, 1922, p. 1.

[30] CME constituency meeting, minutes, February 28, 1923, pp. 6-8

[31] CME board of trustees, minutes, February 7, 1924, p. 4.

[32] CME board of trustees, minutes, July 31, 1958, p. 3.

[33] CME board of trustees, minutes, March 17, 1938, p. 5.

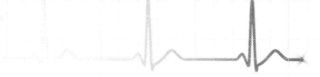

# Chapter 7

# We Have Quality Control!

E fforts to assure quality of health care and to ascertain the qualifications of those involved in its delivery have ancient origins. We find the prototypes in Mosaic law/the Torah, the Code of Hammurabi (Babylonian, c. 1760 B.C.), and the Oath of Hippocrates (Greek, 400 B.C.).

In America political and special interests have often thwarted the standard of health care. A physician's competence in colonial America was usually gained through apprenticeships. However, by the beginning of the nineteenth century the situation began to come under surveillance. In 1901, 23 states demanded more than a diploma to practice medicine, and 37 states required certain credentials for licensure.[1]

A year later, the house of delegates of the American Medical Association and its Council on Medical Education started some serious discussion. The problem? There were too many variations in the education of physicians, the qualification of those seeking licensure, and the different requirements of state boards.

### National Board Examinations

On October 16, 1916, the National Board of Medical Examiners conducted its first examination in Washington, D.C. Sixteen of the 32 applicants qualified. Only five of the 10 who took the test passed.[2] These results underscored the need for regulation.

Dr. Lyle Winslow and Dr. G. Mosser Taylor became the first CME graduates to successfully complete the examinations offered by the National

Board. Both had been members of the class of 1925.[3] Two years later, all of the CME candidates who took part II of the examination passed. In fact, two of them made the honors list.[4]

While attending a session of the Council on Medical Education in Chicago in 1929, Magan reconciled the differences between the National Board of Medical Examiners and the California Board of Medical Examiners. This "equalization" eventually led to legislation that permitted physicians with National Board certificates to register in the state of California.[5]

Obviously, the CME faculty took pride in the performance of these early graduates who took the National Board examinations.[6] Between 1927 and 1930, 16 students received honors in one or more portions of the examination.[7]

In 1927, encouraged by early achievements, Magan proposed that the faculty seriously consider requiring every student to take parts I, II, and III of the National Board examinations.[8] Then, the annual announcement of the School of Medicine (1929-1930) stated that all students entering first-year classes from then on would be required, as part of the curriculum, to pass parts I and II of the National Boards. Part I would be a prerequisite to entering the third year, and part II a prerequisite to entering the fifth year.[9]

The National Board of Medical Examiners helped greatly in establishing "a standard of examinations and certifications of graduates in medicine." Dr. Louis B. Wilson claimed that "the certificate of the National Board is now more widely accepted by licensing bodies than a certificate of passing any other examination in the world."[10]

In retrospect, Dr. John E. Peterson, Sr. (class of 1939) felt that CME benefited in a special way from the developments. The timing of these efforts to raise the standards of medical education and licensure in the United States coincided well with the founding and development of the College of Medical Evangelists. Undoubtedly, it stimulated Loma Linda's continuing "pursuit of excellence":

"It is obvious that both faculty and students were challenged and encouraged by the success of those early graduates who elected to take and pass the examinations of the National Board. It is likely that their success encouraged the faculty to require passing National Board Examinations for promotion. It is also likely that this credential . . . played an important part in helping graduates of a new and relatively unknown school find opportunities for service throughout this country and the world. The remarkable scattering of its graduates within a decade enabled the College of Medical Evangelists to assist the medical mission of Seventh-day Adventists in far corners of the earth. . . . The National Board sought to encourage excellence, and the challenge that it offered to graduates of a small sectarian school most surely played a part in their development and in their ability to participate in a medical mission that has become world wide."[11]

## The Cooperative Plan of Medical Education at CME

CME's constituency heard Newton Evans' report on "The Cooperative Plan of Medical Education" on February 28, 1923. The idea had originated with the dean of the Engineering College at the University of Cincinnati. Evans explained the potential advantages, both to the institution and to its students. The work/study concept had been accepted by other colleges and resulted in an association of schools using the idea. The board of trustees voted to "look with favor" on the innovation.[12] The next day, they voted to place the school on an industrial basis. They requested that Evans and Magan present the concept to the Council on Medical Education for its approval.

From the beginning the Cooperative Plan of Medical Education attempted to make the training of student physicians more practical and effective. Students had more contact with patients, physicians, and nurses. In fact, they actually became economic components of the medical institution. Following consultations with important organizations, CME administrators decided to inaugurate the plan as an educational experiment with the freshman class of 1924.[13]

The Cooperative Plan of Medical Education directed medical students to study one month and to work the next. CME divided each class into two sections. Section I worked while section II studied—then they traded places. Because each student had a replacement in the other half of the class, together they held down one full-time job. Thus student physicians received both practical experience and a living wage in sanitariums, hospitals, laboratories, and physicians' offices throughout Southern California.[14]

To prepare for the Cooperative Plan of Medical Education, medical students arrived at CME two months early. During this time, they studied nursing procedures and the practical aspects of hydrotherapy under Guy R. Kaufmann, a highly respected male nurse. Ora Stains, an educator from the Southern states, coordinated the program and monitored the students on the job. Students and employers greatly appreciated his service.[15]

## The Cooperative Plan of Medical Education at CME (continued)

### How Well Did the Plan Succeed?

The Cooperative Plan of Medical Education proved to be popular with the students. The program had two features designed to enhance the educational value of the work performed. Every month students wrote papers related to their work. Secondly, they participated two times a week in "coordination classes." These meetings were designed to correlate the students' practical experience with the educational curriculum. The curriculum shifted each student to a different type of employment after one year. The administrators made an effort to provide work of progressively increasing technical difficulty and greater responsibility.[16]

Dr. Harold Shryock summarized the results: "For the most part, students enjoyed the change of scene, month by month. On returning to school, after a month's work, the rehearsing of experiences sometimes lasted two or three days before the students got down to solid study. It seemed that each member had some exciting story to tell. . . . By sharing experiences thus, class members broadened their understanding of the practice of medicine. Each student had his own niche to fill while at work, but by comparing his experience with those of his classmates, he could begin to understand the breadth of the medical field."

At the end of each month the students' supervisors completed an employee performance report, which the students reviewed with their coordinator to determine areas of possible future improvement. Since the students in Loma Linda studied six days a week, they completed nine months of studies in six months.[17] The program, however, placed a high demand on CME's faculty. Each class and laboratory session during the first two years had to be repeated.

According to a survey conducted by Newton Evans, the majority of participants felt that the experience benefited them in their comprehension of basic sciences. At the same time, their grasp of instruction during their clinical years improved. Most of the students acknowledged the financial advantages of the program. Indeed, some students were able to earn all of their school expenses. Everyone agreed that the arrangement had no deleterious influence upon their health. Approximately 20 percent of the students reported difficulty in settling down to serious study at the beginning of the month of school work, but the majority, however, maintained that the monthly shifts made it easier for them to study successfully.

### Student Comments on CME's Cooperative Plan of Medical Education

Newton Evans spoke highly of the Cooperative Plan of Medical Education. It combined the science and the art of practicing medicine. Also, it was instrumental in arousing and maintaining the interest of the student physicians, as is noted by their comments:

- "It taught me how to get along with people. Getting among the patients early, talking to them and comforting them, teaches a lot of things that the classroom cannot teach. Contact with leading physicians and observing their methods was a great benefit."

- "A recent graduate of a class-A school told me he had never given a hypodermic injection until after graduation. My experience far exceeds that of this man."

- "It places the student in the medical atmosphere where he meets physicians and patients. This inspires personal confidence and stimulates a desire for study and research."

- "I was more able to comprehend my studies because of having seen how they were applied practically in everyday use, and again having studied certain subjects I understood them more fully when later I saw how they were used. . . . I read upon subjects and studied harder and with more interest after meeting and serving patients in practical work. I have learned to search the literature and summarize my findings in short papers."[18]

The medical superintendent of one hospital reported that his students were well educated and displayed a degree of refinement unknown to the average orderly. The medical students, he said, did work which he had been unable to do until after he had begun his medical practice. The chief medical resident at another large public hospital testified that CME students had learned the secret of success in a medical institution and had acquired the ability to get along "smoothly" with their fellow employees. And, most importantly, they were teachable. Employers (some of whom were initially reluctant to participate) came to consider CME's students indispensable.[19] After graduation, "co-op students" adapted easily to hospital routines. According to Harold Shryock, "they made early progress in developing a degree of self-confidence that worked to their advantage in caring for patients."[20]

Good things, however, eventually come to an end. For whatever reason, the Council on Medical Education came to view the program unfavorably. Therefore, the CME board of trustees voted to discontinue the program at the end of the 1937-1938 school year.[21]

## A New Hospital in Loma Linda

Over the years, by transitioning from a sanitarium to an acute-care hospital, CME served fewer "rest-cure" clients, many of whom were on extended vacations. They cared for more sick patients who had come to learn the secrets of better living. Not only did the medical staff appreciate the variety of interesting cases, but the institution also had to develop new facilities based on patient needs. By the end of the 1920s, a beautiful new Spanish-type structure appeared atop the Hill Beautiful. It combined the features of a sanitarium and hospital under one roof.[22]

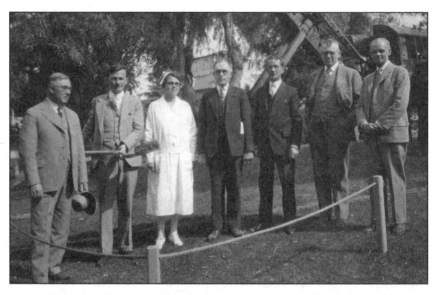

The groundbreaking ceremony for the main section of Loma Linda's new hospital on April 22, 1928.[23] Construction on the 200-foot-long building began that same day.

More than a groundbreaking ceremony, the service became a dedication to "call upon Him who is our Guide and Counselor for His blessings on our efforts."[24] Three days earlier, the board of trustees had invited CME cofounder John Burden, now medical secretary of the Pacific Union Conference, to attend the board meetings. His presence added experience and wisdom to the deliberations.[25]

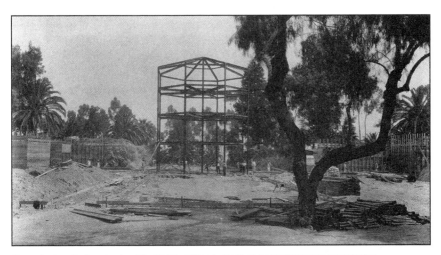

Superstructure for the rotunda of the 1929 addition to the Loma Linda Sanitarium and Hospital.

In October G. H. Curtis, general manager of the Loma Linda Sanitarium, gave a brief report to the board regarding the new sanitarium. Construction, accomplished under a no-debt policy, had advanced only as the institution received funds. Amazingly, it was now apparent that the cost of the building would run considerably under the first estimate. In fact, there were sufficient funds now in sight to complete the building. He hoped that the building could be finished and furnished by the first of February 1929. Then, CME could accommodate the heavy patronage which began every year at about that time.[26]

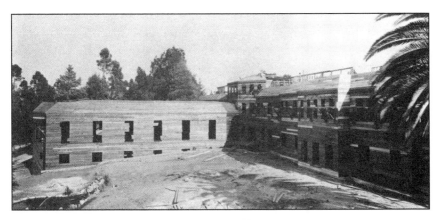

Loma Linda Sanitarium and Hospital under construction, 1929.

TGV1-4

During construction, crews built new roads, redesigned the grounds, and planted 50 different varieties of shrubs, plants, and trees. They even brought in a truckload of desert plants from Arizona. They built a beautiful pond near the main entrance. Set against a background of shrubbery and with water trickling down over the rocks, it looked like a scene in the woods.[27]

Curtis described a special feature of the new hospital: "Provision has recently been made for our hospital patients to have the benefit of outdoor air under a fine new canopy which extends from the extremity of the west wing to the north end of the north wing around a semi-circle, with new cement walks leading thereto. This adds very much to the attractiveness of the hospital grounds, and is a great pleasure to the hospital guests who are still in bed to have this opportunity to enjoy outdoor air, and from which point they can overlook all the beautiful grounds around the sanitarium and the valley and mountain scenery in the distance.[28]

Gardens and landscaping added much to the new "healing place."

"The roadways are being overhauled, new ones being built, electric light fixtures on standards of Spanish type are being erected along the roadways and at the entrance to the grounds and the building—all of these things tending to make the new Loma Linda Sanitarium and its environs a beautiful place."[29]

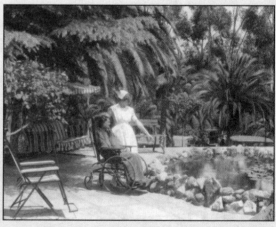

Special effort was taken to make the gardens pleasurable for the patients.

Once again, money came in to fund the huge undertaking. CME administrators acknowledged generous gifts from the General Conference of Seventh-day Adventists, the Pacific Union Conference, the Southern and Southeastern California Conferences, and the Glendale Sanitarium.[30]

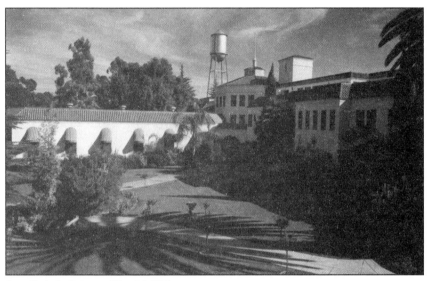

Loma Linda Sanitarium and Hospital, 1930.

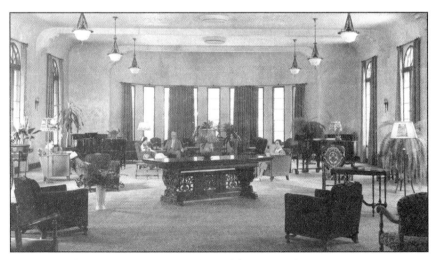

A new parlor in the sanitarium and hospital extended north from the rotunda.

From a practical point of view, the new Loma Linda Sanitarium and Hospital functioned more as a hospital than as an extended care facility. Surgical and obstetrical patients occupied most of the hospital area, and patients with nonsurgical problems occupied the sanitarium area.[31]

As the institution grew, it developed a need for an increased number of physicians trained in the various subspecialties of surgery and medicine. Within one five-year period, the number of qualified specialists with offices in the institution increased 100 percent. The medical staff now reorganized into specialty departments. Of course, the subsequent needs of the departments called for sophisticated equipment. In the 1950s the Department of Radiology had the greatest need. Fortunately, the Ford Foundation donated funds to construct and equip a new Department of Radiology.[32]

### The Great Depression Strikes

Meanwhile in Los Angeles, following the stock market crash of 1929, the Great Depression lowered the occupancy rates to levels never before seen at the White Memorial Hospital. In response, the staff went to great lengths to alleviate the misery. Physicians often accepted flour, chickens, groceries, and other goods as payment for services. A group of registered nurses from the White Memorial Hospital responded with compassion and formed the "Ellen White Nurses" group to serve thousands of poor people in the surrounding community. They donated their time; the hospital provided food; and the county of Los Angeles provided transportation.[33]

The establishment of a new School of Medicine at the University of Southern California in 1928 restored the two-school arrangement at the Los Angeles County Hospital, rebuilding an old partnership. The enormous, new Los Angeles County General Hospital allocated half of its beds to USC and half to CME. Each school presided over its assigned service for each specialty. The Medical Advisory Board of the hospital represented each school.[34] Patient rounds were called "ward walks." On April 15, 1934, Magan delivered the dedicatory address for the new building.[35]

In 1938 the Los Angeles County board of supervisors requested that the University of Southern California and the College of Medical Evangelists supervise medical care at the Los Angeles County General Hospital. The schools then divided the specialty services. This arrangement continued successfully and commendably until 1964 when Loma Linda University began to move its clinical education program to Loma Linda.

"Old timers" remember with great pleasure the many years they shared with the University of Southern California within the walls of the Los Angeles County General Hospital. [36]

[1] W. Carr, "Appointment of State Boards of Medical-Dental Examiners," *Journal of the American Medical Association,* July 6, 1901, 137:6.

[2] N. A. Womack, "Evolution of the National Board of Medical Examiners," *Journal of the American Medical Association,* June 7, 1965, 192:817.

[3] Lucile G. Mallory, "National Board Examinations," *The Medical Evangelist,* July 30, 1925, p. 2.

[4] "National Board," *The Medical Evangelist,* April 28, 1927, p. 4.

[5] Merlin L. Neff, "Taking the Helm," *For God and CME,* p. 268.

[6] Successes in the National Board Examinations were carefully documented in the minutes of faculty meetings and in "News Notes" in the *Medical Evangelist.*

[7] "News Notes," *The Medical Evangelist,* April 28, 1927; June 14, 1928; May 23, 1929; August 1, 1929; and May 15, 1930. John E. Peterson, M.D., "CME-LLU and the National Board," *Diamond Memories,* p. 140.

[8] Dr. Magan proposed that the National Board Examinations parts I, II, and III be taken at the end of the second, fourth, and fifth years of medicine, respectively. Discussion followed, but the board made no decision at that time. See CME faculty minutes, July 20, 1927, p. 158.

[9] *CME 21st Annual Announcement,* 1929-1930, p. 38. Today, passing part I of the National Boards is a prerequisite to entering the third year and passing part II is required for graduation. (John E. Peterson, M.D., "CME-LLU and the National Board," *Diamond Memories,* p. 140. Confirmed by Loretta Miyasato, August 23, 2004.)

[10] L. B. Wilson, M.D., "The Work of the National Board of Medical Examiners During its First Quarter Century," *Diplomate,* 12:161, 1940 (quoted from W. L. Rodman).

[11] John E. Peterson, M.D., "CME-LLU and the National Board," *Diamond Memories,* p. 141.

[12] Newton G. Evans, M.D., "Cooperative Plan in Medical Education—Four Years Experience," *The Medical Evangelist,* January 3, 1929, p. 1.

[13] *CME Annual Announcement,* July 1924, p. 27. The CME administrators counseled with Henry S. Pritchett of the Carnegie Foundation and others, including the State Board of Medical Examiners of California and the Council on Medical Education.

[14] Evans, p. 2.

[15] Harold Shryock, "The Cooperative Plan," *Diamond Memories,* p. 130.

[16] Evans, p.2, Shryock, p.130.

[17] Shryock, p.130.

[18] Evans, pp. 2, 3.

[19] *Ibid.* After the first four years, 467 students (including dietetics students) had been employed by 33 hospitals, seven sanitariums, 17 physicians' offices, 22 clinical laboratories (including various hospital laboratories), and X-ray laboratories.

[20] Shryock, p. 132.

[21] CME board of trustees, minutes, April 12, 1937, p. 2.

[22] Clarence A. Miller, "The Loma Linda San," *Diamond Memories*, p. 22.

[23] Participants at the groundbreaking ceremony included (left to right): Comptroller F. E. Corson, who acted as master of ceremonies; Medical Director Dan Burgeson, M.D., who lifted the first spade of soil; director of the School of Nursing, Mrs. Daisy E. Walton, R.N.; Business Manager G. H. Curtis, who delivered the principal address of the day; Chaplain S.T. Hare, who offered prayer; dean of the Los Angeles Division, Newton G. Evans, M.D.; and dean of the Loma Linda Division, Edward H. Risley, M.D. This hospital building is now known as Nichol Hall.

[24] *The Medical Evangelist*, May 3, 1928, p. 2.

[25] *Ibid.*, April 19, 1928, p. 3.

[26] CME board of trustees, minutes, October 18, 1928, p. 2.

[27] *The Medical Evangelist*, October 18, 1928, pp. 1, 2.

[28] *Ibid.*, p. 2.

[29] *Ibid.*, p. 2; and March 7, 1929, p. 2.

[30] Keynote speech by G. H. Curtis, general manager of the Loma Linda Sanitarium, during groundbreaking ceremony on Sunday, April 29, 1928. The text was reproduced in *The Medical Evangelist,* May 3, 1928, p. 2.

[31] Miller, p. 22.

[32] *Ibid.*, p. 24.

[33] *Hands of Healing in the City of Angels—90 Years, 1913-2003* (Los Angeles, California; White Memorial Medical Center), p. 4; Keld J. Reynolds, Ph.D., "Accreditation Victory," *Outreach*, p. 41.

[34] Walter E. Macpherson, M.D., "The County," *Diamond Memories,* p. 77. Having outgrown its former facilities on Mission Road, the Los Angeles County Hospital moved into its huge present structure in 1932.

[35] Walter E. Macpherson, M.D., "Percy Tilson Magan, M.D.," *Diamond Memories*, p. 168. Helen Eastman Martin, M.D., *The History of the Los Angeles County Hospital (1878-1968)* (Los Angeles, California: University of Southern California Press, 1979), p. 117.

[36] Walter E. Macpherson, "The County," *Diamond Memories*, p. 78.

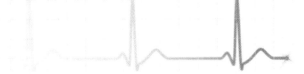

# Chapter 8

# Adventures in Management:
# An Old Challenge Reappears

In 1934 CME administrators became anxious when the American Medical Association's Council on Medical Education announced plans to resurvey every school of medicine in America. They intended to significantly reduce the number of schools. Some feared that the religious nature of CME would be a handicap. Could the school retain its class A rating? Magan explained the problem to church leaders. He described it as being "the most momentous undertaking" of its kind which has ever been launched:

"No similar piece of work has ever been done and expectations run high and wide as to what it will accomplish. There can be no question but what the medical powers-that-be have big things in their heads. They have openly announced that there is a large difference today between the best medical colleges and the poorest in our land, as there was in the early years of this century when they cut the number of medical schools almost exactly in half, putting 50 percent of these institutions out of business. These men are firmly of the opinion that some medical schools will have to go. I do not think they have us particularly in mind. . . . However, I do realize that when it comes to buildings and equipment and to the size of teaching personnel that we are almost hopelessly behind practically every other medical college in the land."[1]

Magan used the imminent inspection as a means of leverage to secure more funds from the board for much-needed buildings and equipment: "Of course, if they see that we are doing things to improve our building and equipment items, they will be much more inclined to do leniency with us than otherwise."[2]

The Council on Medical Education evaluated every school of medicine in the United States and Canada. On the Loma Linda campus the North Laboratory was condemned. Earthquakes had weakened the cement walls to such an extent that engineers declared the building unsafe. The loss of the North Laboratory was a terrible blow to the institution. Furthermore, the secretary of the Council on Medical Education told Magan that CME had to invest in more teachers, better teacher training, and additional buildings. Finally, he asked, "Can you raise half a million dollars?"[3]

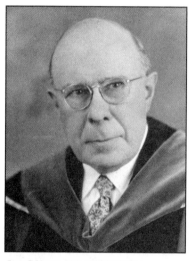

Percy T. Magan, M.D. (1867-1947)

By the time of the denomination's 1934 Autumn Council, Magan had secured appropriations of half a million dollars to prepare the school for inspection. Later he returned to Chicago and informed the secretary that the school had met his recommendation. "Well, Doctor, I have seen our bishops and the $500,000 has been provided."[4]

The secretary leaped out of his seat, embraced Magan, and exclaimed, "You have wonderful bishops! You have wonderful bishops! I didn't believe there was that much money in the country in these hard days for a small and hard-pressed medical school!"

The man invited Magan to his home for dinner that night. "His wife met us at the door, grasped both my hands in hers, and in a voice ringing with emotion said, 'Oh, Dr. Magan, I am so glad, so glad, so glad!' Surely the Lord has dealt mercifully with us. Blessed and blessed be His holy name."[5]

This incident provides insight into Magan's character and influence within the church and the medical community. Magan was a skilled warrior for CME, persuading the General Conference of Seventh-day Adventists to once again financially support its flagship institution. Because of Magan's influence, the AMA official and his wife were privately pulling for CME. Seeing the result as yet another act of Providence, Magan gave the credit to the One who continued to intervene on behalf of CME.

## Fulfilling AMA's Requirements

With additional support from alumni and friends, CME built three new basic science buildings in Loma Linda between 1936 and 1940. During that time period, the faculty grew to be the largest in CME's history. Employees numbered almost a thousand. The institution also built a new, multistory White Memorial Hospital in Los Angeles. Classes had grown from 10 to almost 130.[6]

On March 8, 1936, the inspection committee met with Magan at the Biltmore Hotel in Los Angeles. For four hours, they fired questions at him "with all the speed and precision and accuracy of machine-gun fire."[7]

When the examiners visited Loma Linda, the group sat down to eat in the Loma Linda Sanitarium dining room. Magan asked Risley to say grace. Impressed by this prayer, Dr. Herman Weiskotten said, "This is the first meal to which I have sat down since I left home where the blessing was asked." The examiners also commented on the spirit of sacrifice that permeated the faculty and alumni—many of whom had become missionaries to India, Africa, and China.

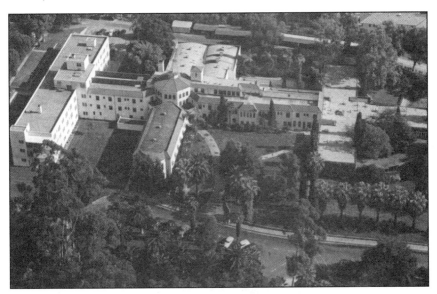

The east wing of the Loma Linda Sanitarium and Hospital (far left) was built in 1949. Two of the original buildings, Southwest Cottage and Large Cottage, were razed for this addition. This facility eventually became a 186-bed community hospital.

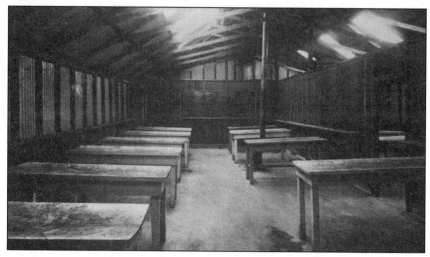

The Anatomy Laboratory rested on a cement slab near San Timoteo Creek. Medical students quickly dubbed it "Jericho." The building was well hidden by a surrounding orange grove.[9]

Some of the criticisms, of course, were valid, especially those regarding teaching methods and the shortage of personnel in some departments. In

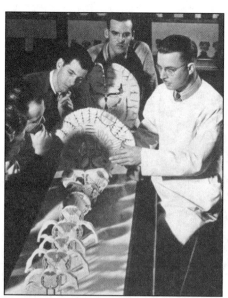

Harold Shryock, M.D., teaching Neuro-anatomy at CME.

general, however, the school made a deep and positive impression. While driving back to the hotel on the last day of the inspection, Dr. M. W. Ireland remarked, "Well, I'm hypnotized by that place!"

As the gentlemen said goodbye, they declared, "This has been the greatest day since we started out on this work. We have enjoyed every minute of it!"[8]

The AMA closed or placed on probation several wealthy medical schools—schools that were much better known than CME. Eventually, however, CME was awarded another class A rating. The spiritual emphasis had, indeed, made a favorable impression.

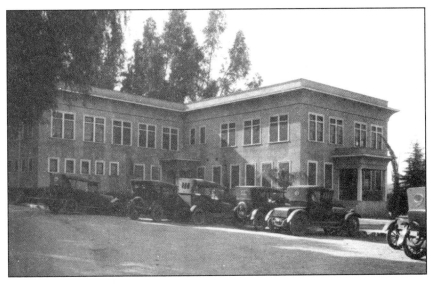

The new building, named South Laboratory, eventually housed the School of Tropical and Preventive Medicine and became the first home of the School of Public Health. According to Harold Shryock, M.D., this parking lot once accommodated every automobile in Loma Linda.

## Bureaucratic Compassion?

In 1939 an unusual request came to the board that reflected the institution's accreditation controversy 22 years earlier when the school had only a C rating. The State Board in North Carolina denied Dr. Edna Patterson, a 1917 graduate of CME, permission to take its examination. If she were to retake the senior year now that CME had the A rating, however, North Carolina would reconsider. Not only did the board vote to allow her to retake her senior year, but it also specified that it would be without further cost to her.[10]

---

[1] Percy T. Magan, M.D., "The Vision Undimmed by Shadows," *For God and CME*, p. 283.
[2] Magan, pp. 283, 284.
[3] Magan, "Report of the President," *The Medical Evangelist,* February 15, 1940, p. 5.
[4] Even though the Seventh-day Adventist Church has no bishops, Magan used termi-

nology that would help the secretary realize that top-level church administrators had again come to CME's rescue.

[5] *Ibid.*

[6] *Ibid.*

[7] The AMA Inspection Committee included Dr. Herman Weiskotten and Surgeon General M. W. Ireland. See Magan, *For God and CME*, p. 286.

[8] Magan, *Ibid.*, p. 287; letter to C. H. Watson and J. L. Shaw, March 13, 1936.

[9] CME board of trustees, minutes, January 5, 1913, p. 127.

[10] CME board of trustees, minutes, September 7, 1939, p. 3. Furthermore, the board asked Dr. Walter E. Macpherson to obtain detailed information from North Carolina regarding just what special subjects Dr. Patterson would need to take so that there would be no question of her receiving recognition at that time.

# Chapter 9:

# The Los Angeles Campus

Following two years of intense basic sciences instruction, student physicians moved to Los Angeles for clinical training. In Loma Linda students focused on educational activities. In Los Angeles they centered on the patient. As the patient became the textbook and formal lectures gave way to individual instruction, the students became participants in patient care. The White Memorial Hospital symbolized the highest standards of medical practice and became the students' educational and spiritual home for the latter portion of their training.[1]

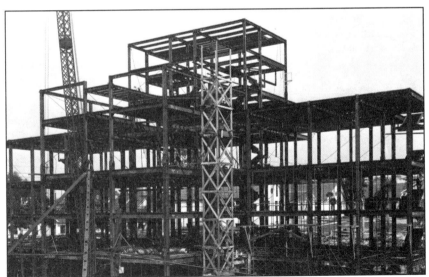

The 1937 addition to the White Memorial Hospital under construction.

In 1937, to meet ever-increasing demands, CME dedicated a new $330,000 concrete-and-steel wing to the White Memorial Hospital. The seven-story, 190-bed wing was the first earthquake-resistant hospital structure in California.[2] In 1953 the school again expanded with a new $2.5-million wing. It added 128,800 square feet of floor space and increased the bed capacity to 300.

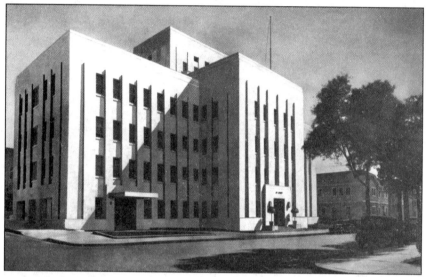

The completed structure.

By 1960, 300 physicians and scores of nurses and technicians who had trained at CME were serving or had served in foreign medical mission posts around the world. Their contribution to the health and welfare of thousands of people can never be fully measured. In addition to their impact in foreign countries, CME touched thousands of lives in Los Angeles. Since its humble beginnings in 1913, the CME staff and students had delivered 35,000 babies. The institution scheduled 140,000 outpatient appointments annually. And since the White Memorial Hospital opened in 1918, more than 200,000 patients had been admitted.[3]

But statistics and structures didn't tell the most important part of the story. The institution provided a Christian environment where teachers could teach, where students could learn, where students and staff could practice the healing arts together, and where patients could experience wholeness from a ministry of healing. It is a story of God's work by individuals for individuals.

## Not Enough Space

By 1941, 2,500 patients crowded the White's dispensary every week. These people could not afford to pay a private physician but were not financially eligible for care by existing city and county agencies. Thankfully, they benefited from the clinic's unique efforts to provide access to medical advice and treatment. Without aid from any philanthropic group (except appropriations from the General Conference of Seventh-day Adventists), the White Memorial Clinic had become one of the largest of its kind in America, serving 164,000 patients in 1940.

In addition CME maintained a home maternity service whose staff delivered

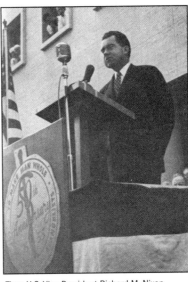

Then U.S. Vice President Richard M. Nixon spoke at dedication ceremonies at White Memorial Hospital (March 1955) as part of the institution's 50th anniversary celebration.[4]

more than 50 infants a month. The White Memorial Clinic offered patients prenatal, home delivery, and postnatal care for a minimum fee.[5]

## World War II Impacts CME: The 47th General Hospital

Soon after the close of World War I, some of the younger physicians at CME proposed that the college organize a Seventh-day Adventist-staffed, stand-by military hospital as a gesture of cooperation with the United States government. Magan, dean of the School of Medicine, very much favored the idea. Therefore, he negotiated with officers of the Ninth Corps Area of the United States Army in San Francisco to establish the 47th General Hospital of the United States Army Medical Corps.[6]

CME officially organized the hospital in 1926 when Newton Evans became its commanding officer and assumed the rank of Lieutenant Colonel in the Reserves. Shortly thereafter, Dr. Cyril B. Courville (class of 1925) became the head of the 47th General Hospital. Courville's consistent devotion to the hospital built it into a highly efficient unit. Its staff included physicians, nurses, administrative officers, and physical therapists. The hospital included all of the medical and surgical services required by Army regulations. Its reserve officers spent a few days each year in active military training.[7]

## The Medical Cadet Corps

Training Seventh-day Adventist youth to be "medics" instead of combat soldiers became a worthy cause. Officers of the 47th General Hospital helped to train young men who were not otherwise medically oriented in the popular Medical Cadet Corps. Participants then offered needed services to their country without violating the church's noncombatant position. The Medical Cadet Corps attracted favorable attention both from church members and the surgeon general's office.[8]

In 1940 the United States Army Medical Corps and the United States surgeon general proposed that CME reorganize the Army's 47th General Hospital. This was the Medical Reserve Corps hospital that CME had organized but not activated during World War I.[9]

The General Conference had approved of the Medical Reserve Corps Hospital at the time of its inception. Now it fostered frank discussion. Many felt that the 47th General Hospital, manned entirely by Seventh-day Adventists from CME, would create goodwill. It could demonstrate to anyone who might criticize CME's noncombatant position that the institution was willing to conscientiously support the war efforts in their own way. Furthermore, Sabbath observance and dietary considerations could be accommodated.[10]

CME named a temporary committee to study and recommend assignment of personnel. Then, in case of mobilization, the calling of medical officers would not seriously impact the operations of the School of Medicine. The board also expressed appreciation to Courville for his untiring efforts in keeping the 47th General Hospital alive. The advantages of the plan would assuredly further the denomination's relationship with the United States military.[11]

## World War II Becomes a United States Responsibility

In January 1941 Magan gave a potentially troubling report. The Army was rapidly enlarging its medical program and was in dire need of staffing other units. This created complications for CME because the military was rapidly pulling officers out of the 47th General Hospital.[12]

The next year, in 1942, CME permitted the United States Army and Navy to interview students in the preclinical Loma Linda Division and recruit for the Medical Reserve. Students would be able to complete their medical course without the probability of being drafted. After prayerful study, however, board members felt that some student physicians might never be called. In that case, membership in the reserves would subject them to immediate service upon completion of their medical course. The board urged CME to advise its students to wait until they were drafted to join the reserves.[13]

In 1943 the United States activated the 47th General Hospital and Colonel Ben E. Grant, M.D. (class of 1920), became commandant. Because of his devotion and many years of service, Courville was expected to command the hospital if it were ever activated in wartime, but unfortunately, he was unable to assume these duties because of health reasons.[14] The S. S. *West Point* transported the 47th General Hospital to the South Pacific where CME officers helped construct the facility in Milne Bay[15] at the southern tip of Papua, New Guinea.

**Wartime Changes**

During World War II the United States War Department virtually commandeered America's medical schools to increase the number of physicians available for the war effort. To assure itself of having a continuous supply of young physicians to serve as medical officers in the United States military, the War Department implemented its "Accelerated Program." Beginning July 1, 1943, CME cooperated in the interest of national security.[16]

Under this new program, everything sped up. CME eliminated vacations and started classes every nine months. It reduced its medical curriculum from four years to three and increased its class size from 75 students to 96. The freshman class started on July 1 instead of in September.

Most of the male students were of military age and had been deferred from active military service as a courtesy by their respective draft boards. Now, according to the new regulations, they had to join the United States military.[17] Then, the military assumed authority for placing medical students in the nation's medical schools.[18] The government announced that it would assign medical school applicants randomly from Washington, D.C.

This development had the makings of a disaster. CME projected that the program would deteriorate with alcohol-using, smoking, nonvegetarian individuals on campus who would be totally ignorant about Loma Linda's conservative, religious ideals. A crisis loomed!

The board of trustees sent Dr. Walter E. Macpherson, dean of the School of Medicine, to Washington, D.C., where he met Colonel Walter S. Jensen, M.D. (class of 1924). One of Macpherson's former classmates, Jensen opened doors for the visitor. Finally, Macpherson saw a Colonel White. As he presented CME's problem to White, a soldier entered his office and handed the colonel a communiqué. The message was exhilarating! White had just been promoted to the rank of brigadier general! Caught up in the excitement of his promotion, White promptly drafted details of how the plan to assist Loma Linda might work.[19] Providence did work in a spectacular and practical way. CME became the only school of medicine in America allowed to choose its own students, starting with those about to be assigned to other schools.[20]

In the summer of 1943 the board of trustees approved the installation of Army Specialized Training Program (ASTP) Number 3934 on both campuses. CME dedicated its special Loma Linda unit on September 15, complete with military headquarters in the new men's dormitory. As a symbol of coauthority, the major in charge of the military cadre of two lieutenants and four enlisted men requested to have an office next to Dean Harold Shryock's office in the Pathology Building. (Harold Shryock was at that time acting dean of the Loma Linda Division.)

## Learning to Live Together

The relationship was imagined to be one of host and guest—CME being the host, and the new army unit being the guest. Sometimes, however, the "guest" tried to dominate the "host." The first army officer incorrectly assumed that he commanded all campus facilities. Compromises in the scheduling of classes and laboratory sessions in order to accommodate military instructions, marching drills, and gas mask drills eased tensions. Several months later the military promoted that officer and replaced him with a businessman from the Army Reserves. The new commandant cooperated with CME administrators and honored the religious convictions he encountered.

CME observed Saturday, the Sabbath, as a day of freedom from classes and military activities on campus. The military honored CME's preference for a vegetarian diet. The cadre of military officers also complied with CME's prohibitions against the use of alcoholic beverages and tobacco. Occasions of disputed authority were few and were not disruptive. The United States Navy inducted a few of the students who traveled off campus to Long Beach for military instruction and drills.

Financial rewards were not to be ignored. The United States military issued uniforms and paid tuition. Students received a financial stipend greater than the wages of an unskilled laborer. Married men received even greater remuneration. A father received additional funds for each child. Participants had access to discounted goods at the "PX" in Daniells Hall as well as prospects for future veteran's benefits. Some faculty observed that students fared better financially than did their teachers. At the conclusion of their training, the new physicians became commissioned officers. Some administrators considered these highly unusual circumstances to be providential.

## Academic Strictures

Unfortunately, the nine-month cycle did not match the 12-month cycle of the Adventist senior colleges, where most prospective medical students took their prerequisite courses. Premed students in those schools sometimes had to wait several months before starting CME's next freshman class. During these months of waiting, local Selective Service System boards occasionally attempted to induct these students into the military, even though they had already been admitted to CME. Harold Shryock had to negotiate with local boards and sometimes appeal to the appropriate state board for review. On at least one occasion Harold Shryock had to appeal to the National Selective Service System in Washington, D.C., in order to obtain a temporary deferment for one of his students.

Ongoing military interactions complicated administrative responsibilities. Filling faculty vacancies became virtually impossible. At this time the armed forces tried to induct Harold Shryock. Fortunately, because of his position as dean of the Loma Linda Division, the military deferred him from active service.

## Postwar Recovery

By the end of World War II the cadre of military officers had endeared themselves to CME by their cooperation and sympathetic attitudes: "And we missed them," Harold Shryock said. CME had graduated four classes in three years. By now, everybody was tired, both the students and the faculty. In 1947 the college restored its 12-month curriculum and easily resumed class schedules and course sequences that had been altered to accommodate the military program. A welcome peace replaced the long-lasting uncertainty among students and faculty.

The United States military benefited from CME's willingness to serve as a Christian witness for the church. Both the 47th General Hospital and medics who had been trained in the Medical Cadet Corps received high commendation for serving valiantly in the South Pacific. More than 500 CME alumni saw military service during World War II. Included in this number were physicians serving outside of the 47th General Hospital. Many were decorated—the Army Silver Star, the Bronze Star Medal, the Citation for Meritorious Achievement, and the Citation for Legion of Merit—because of the quality of services they performed. Some became prisoners of war, and some died in service to their country.[21]

Representative of those who made the ultimate sacrifice was Dr. Edward Curtin (class of 1941), who died when enemy forces bombed and strafed his PT boat. A lieutenant in the Navy's Medical Corps, Curtin was assigned to a squadron of PT boats operating near New Britain. Although medical officers did not customarily accompany PT boats on patrol, Curtin thought his services might be needed there most. After being hit, he directed the care of others, even as he lay dying. In a spirit of self-sacrifice and courage, he insisted that aid be administered to others first. For his bravery in the line of duty, the United States military awarded Curtin Navy and Marine Corps medals of honor posthumously.[22]

---

[1] *The March of CME*, 1953, vol. 3, p. 45.

[2] *Hands of Healing in The City of Angels—90 Years, 1913-2003*, White Memorial Medical Center, p. 4.

[3] Erwin J. Remboldt, "Serving the Sick of Los Angeles," *Signs of the Times*, June 1960, pp. 12, 31.

[4] "Vice-president Richard Nixon Praises SDA Medical Work and Workers," *The Voice*

*of CME Employees,* April 1955, p. 3. For most of his life Dr. George Akers has been called Nixon's "double." They met on this occasion, and Nixon said, "We *do* look alike!" On one occasion, Akers was taken to be Nixon at the entrance to Camp David, Maryland. The breach of security was horrendous. An account of that event is now found in the Nixon Library, California.

[5] *The March of CME* (Los Angeles, California: Student-Faculty Association of the College of Medical Evangelists, 1941), pp. 103, 104.

[6] Harold Shryock, M.D., "The War Years," *Diamond Memories,* p. 104.

[7] *Ibid.*

[8] *Ibid.*

[9] CME board of trustees, minutes, May 16, 1940, p. 4. This report was presented to the CME Board by Drs. Macpherson and Flaiz.

[10] *Ibid.,* p. 5.

[11] *Ibid.,* p. 6.

[12] *Ibid.,* January 16, 1941, p. 3

[13] *Ibid.,* February 2, 1942, p. 13.

[14] Shryock, p. 104.

[15] *Ibid.,* p. 106.

[16] CME board of trustees, minutes, February 26, 1942, p. 6; August 26, 1943, p. 9.

[17] *Ibid.;* Carrol S. Small, M.D., "Curriculum," *Diamond Memories,* p. 122.

[18] CME board of trustees, minutes, August 26, 1943, p. 9.

[19] Shryock, p. 108.

[20] CME board of trustees, minutes, January 25, 1951, p. 7.

[21] *Ibid.*

[22] *Ibid.*

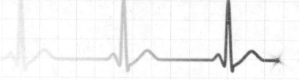

Chapter 10:

# Consolidation:
# The Controversy of the Century

At the beginning of the twentieth century, medical education authorities required formal education in both basic sciences and clinical experience. In response the majority of medical schools in America taught basic sciences on their main campus in a rural setting and clinical education at a large hospital in a convenient nearby city. Examples included the University of California at Berkeley, Stanford University, Cornell University, and the College of Medical Evangelists.[1]

In 1936 and again in 1939 the Council on Medical Education of the American Medical Association and the Executive Council of the Association of American Medical Colleges referred to CME's two-campus division as a handicap. Subsequent reports in 1951, 1954, and 1958 all discussed the disadvantages inherent with teaching courses 60 miles apart and recommended unification of the School of Medicine.[2] This idea would evolve into a long, slow controversy, the likes of which no one could imagine at the time.

### The Proposal

In 1946 the board first discussed the possibility of moving the clinical division of CME to Loma Linda. Macpherson clearly indicated his willingness to have the entire school located in Loma Linda. At this time, however, he also believed that the area did not have a large enough population to provide the estimated number of patients that would be needed for clinicals. Nevertheless, the board considered the possibility to be of such significance that it appointed a 21-person committee to study the issue.[3] Here began a long succession of committees—large ones—to explore the whole range of pros and cons surrounding this decision.

The next year (1947) a constituency meeting in Loma Linda also discussed the possibility of moving CME's clinical program back to Loma Linda. Ellen White reportedly had stated that Seventh-day Adventist medical institutions would be more successful outside of big cities.[4]

The Los Angeles Division (affectionately known as "The City") had been established because of a perceived lack of potential patients in the early days around the Loma Linda Division (affectionately known as "The Farm"). Los Angeles provided an abundance of patients for the clinical education of medical and nursing students. In addition to the White Memorial Hospital, the affiliated 19-story Los Angeles County General Hospital allocated half of its 3,400 beds[5] to the University of Southern California and half to CME. It was the largest acute-care hospital in the world, under one roof.

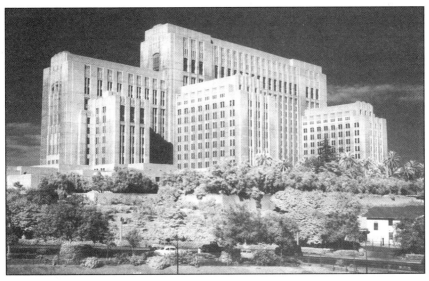

The Los Angeles County General Hospital opened in 1933.

Maxine Atteberry, dean of the School of Nursing, assessed several facets of the situation:

**1. Internationalism.** The contrast between the two campuses was enormous. Loma Linda provided a country atmosphere and slower–paced activities. Patients were mostly white, middle-class Americans. Many were long-term patients, and some returned time after time. The area was peaceful and quiet, with orange groves, farms, pepper trees, and palms surrounding the campus. Loma Linda did accommodate acute medical and surgical patients, but the hectic life of an acute hospital was minimized by the country surroundings and by the number of "sanitarium" patients who found the place restful and restorative.

The White Memorial Hospital, on the other hand, was located in the midst of a large foreign population—a Russian colony lived a few blocks to the west, and a large Jewish community was located just east of the Boyle Avenue location. North and south were mixtures of many races and ethnic groups. Many Mexican-Americans, among a mixture of other races and ethnic groups, lived to the north and south of the hospital, adding interest to the throng who came to the clinic and hospital for medical care.[6]

**2. OB/GYN.** The White's dispensary provided rich learning experiences for CME's students in the area of OB/GYN. Sometimes outpatient services included home deliveries in the surrounding community, where senior nursing students joined junior and senior medical students to provide "outside OB." Because few students had cars, they traveled by streetcar or walked, sometimes traveling through the slums and ghettos of East Los Angeles at night.[7]

**3. The Los Angeles County General Hospital.** A landmark with 76 standard wards on its acute unit alone, the Los Angeles County General Hospital had become CME's "third campus." Student physicians spent their junior year there. Student nurses spent a part of their senior year there. In 1957 CME had almost 50 paid employees working at "the County," and they were just as busy as any employee working on the other two campuses.[8]

**4. Collegiality.** In her book *History of the Los Angeles County Hospital,* Dr. Helen Martin wrote: "It is noteworthy that the schools of medicine of the University of Southern California and the College of Medical Evangelists functioned throughout their years of association without major controversy. This was particularly true during the period when Drs. Raulston (USC) and Macpherson (CME) were associated as [representatives] of their respective schools. Drs. Raulston and Macpherson were real gentlemen, in the finest tradition of the word. This quality did much to prevent the fighting and feuding which has occurred at many county hospitals shared by several medical schools, where frank hostility, aggressive competition, or cold separateness have developed."[9]

**5. The "Inland Empire" Prospers.** In early 1951, as the population of the Riverside-San Bernardino-Redlands metropolitan area continued to grow, the board authorized Macpherson to conduct another investigation and report at its April 11 meeting regarding the feasibility of moving the campus. His report called the feasibility "questionable" and indicated that further study would be needed to come to a sound conclusion. Because a Ramona Boulevard site in Alhambra was, at that time, still a viable alternative, the board appointed yet another committee to study the issues.[10] So, the multiplication of committees went on.

### Consolidation Is the Ideal

Everyone agreed that CME's operations, which included duplication of offices and long commutes, should be consolidated on one campus to make the School of Medicine more cost effective and logistically sound. However, deciding on which one would be the best was the question.

An inspection in November 1951, by the Council on Medical Education of the American Medical Association and the Association of American Medical Colleges, resulted in a recommendation that the board of trustees give serious consideration to uniting the school on the Los Angeles campus. On April 6, 1953, representatives of the council and the association met with a committee of CME and General Conference representatives to reiterate their previous recommendations to consolidate in Los Angeles.[11]

A few days later (April 9-10) the board of trustees acknowledged the feasibility of operating the School of Medicine in Los Angeles. Nonetheless, they appointed yet *another* fact-finding commission to determine the possibility of operating an accredited school entirely on the Loma Linda campus.[12]

In an editorial in the Seventh-day Adventist church paper, Francis D. Nichol announced that the Ellen G. White Publications Office had provided copies of everything Ellen White had written regarding the church's medical work in general and Loma Linda in particular. In a sincere effort to seek the will of God, he reported that church leaders had studied these works diligently and prayerfully.[13] Throughout her writings, frequent references to Loma Linda caused a majority of the commission members to conclude that the school *should not be consolidated in Los Angeles.*

Yet, following weeks of exhaustive study, the commission concluded that it would be financially and professionally impractical to conduct even a small medical school solely on the Loma Linda campus. Furthermore, in the process it would probably lose its accreditation by the AMA. Members also expressed hope that eventually a strong group of clinicians in Loma Linda might open the door to conducting the entire curriculum of the School of Medicine in Loma Linda.[14]

### Sidestepping the Issue

On September 20, 1953, after a thorough study and considerable discussion, the board voted "that if the school must be located on one campus, it should be Loma Linda." Because of the expense involved, however, and the possibility of reduction in capacity, they recommended that CME continue operations on both campuses.[15]

That year the White Memorial Clinic was the largest privately owned outpatient dispensary west of Chicago, with an average of 550 patients a day. Except for services available at the county hospital, CME served more outpatients than any other institution in southern California. Students rotated among nearly 50 separate subclinics, each devoted to specific diseases. The clinic served those who were unable to pay for private medical care, regardless of race, color, creed, or nationality[16] How could CME give this up?

Ultimately, the decision would be taken out of the board's hands. In 1958 accrediting authorities again opposed the two-campus arrangement. Instead of *recommending* consolidation on one campus, they *required* it. One board member called it "a polite ultimatum."[17] By 1959 CME had become the only school of medicine in America to operate on two campuses.[18]

### The Two Parties Meet, Head-on

Would CME consolidate in Loma Linda or in Los Angeles?

The basic science faculty in Loma Linda favored Loma Linda. The volunteer Los Angeles clinical faculty favored Los Angeles. The church constituency and most of the university councilors favored Loma Linda. The board and CME administrators were split. Both sides were adamant, and both sides were sincere. Opposing views claimed that consolidation in Los Angeles would alienate the church constituency, which had been so supportive over the years. Consolidation in Loma Linda, on the other hand, would kill the School of Medicine. With an inadequate number of patients around Loma Linda, some argued, CME would be unable to maintain its accreditation.

### Champions of the Consolidation Cause

Because his term was about to expire, Glenn Calkins addressed a six-page letter to his fellow board members expressing his feelings on the matter. He reiterated the commission's conclusion that heeding the counsels of Ellen White and acting in harmony with the guiding principles of Christian education, as set forth in her writings, had brought CME to its present state of development.

Calkins also cited the conclusion of the 1953 Autumn Council of the church—if the school had to be located on one campus, it should be Loma Linda. This would be in harmony with the intent and purpose in establishing the school, according to Ellen White's counsel. He was greatly disturbed when he heard a fellow board member at the December 18, 1958, meeting say, "All religious discussion should be kept out of the question and decisions made solely in the light of present–day scientific facts and needs."

### Are We Overlooking the Spiritual Component?

Calkins stated his case forcefully: "I immediately challenged that statement, for I believe the medical school was established under divine instruction given through the messenger of the Lord, and that as the result, 'religious discussion' of any of its problems is not only right and proper, but is definitely needed now as we face this grave crisis.... The real question before us, as I saw it, was whether we accept that instruction, or on the other hand are we to be governed entirely by counsel from worldly organizations. In short, do we accept literally the Spirit of Prophecy as divinely given instruction, or do we virtually reject it by avoiding any religious discussion of the question?

"It appears to me that unless we are ready to give consideration to and follow that instruction, we might as well think of closing the Medical School, for what valid reason do we have in asking the denomination to continue to pour in tremendous sums of money each year to support a school simply to compete with scientific schools of the world."

Calkins confronted his colleagues in a powerful conclusion: "Looking at the question from purely a human viewpoint, it would seem almost impossible to unite on either campus now because of the teaching and financial problems involved. However if the college is required to take steps looking forward to uniting the two campuses how dare we disregard the plain instructions from God? Should we fail to follow the counsel of the Lord I am fearful for the future of our school."[19]

In a five-page letter to Walter P. Elliott, chair of the board of trustees, Dr. Mervin G. Hardinge advised him to look at CME's memorable heritage: "The College of Medical Evangelists is an institution established in faith by God through human instrumentalities. The decisions that must now be made are no more difficult than those which confronted our pioneers some fifty years ago. As we, God's servants, act in faith in accord with His will, the answers to the problems will be given."[20]

As a member of numerous committees, Hardinge was deeply involved in preparing materials that showed trends in medical education supporting Ellen White's counsels for the denomination to conduct a school of medicine in Loma Linda.[21] Meanwhile, board members received passionate input from people on *both* sides of the issue.

Willis J. Hackett, president of the Atlantic Union Conference, expressed his opinion to Dr. Bernard D. Briggs, chair of the Department of Anesthesiology and also a board member: "If we only had the Urim and the Thummim of the Old Testament tabernacle service to guide us, it would be helpful."[22]

Briggs referred to a "Red Sea experience" and applied a quotation from Ellen White's writings to support his straightforward position, saying that it would be presumptuous for the school to consolidate in Los Angeles.[23] "There is a great similarity between our history and that of the children of Israel. . . . The voice of the Lord bidding His faithful ones 'go forward' frequently tries their faith to the uttermost. But if they should defer obedience till every shadow of uncertainty was removed from their understanding, and there remained no risk of failure or defeat, they would never move on at all. Those who think it impossible for them to yield to the will of God and have faith in His promises until all is made clear and plain before them will never yield at all. Faith is not certainty of knowledge; it is 'the substance of things hoped for, the evidence of things not seen'. . . . 'Go forward' should be the Christian's watchword."[24]

## Some Helpful Changes

By 1958 demographic changes in the Loma Linda area answered some of the problems encountered earlier. The population of Riverside and San Bernardino counties had grown from 450,000 to 735,000 between 1950 and 1958, and it was estimated to reach 1.25 million by 1966. In 1960 the two nearby county hospitals were about to complete multimillion-dollar modernization programs, increasing bed capacities to 1,100. Both hospitals would be available to provide clinical experience. Moreover, contrary to earlier predictions, the School of Dentistry had an overabundance of patients.[25]

On February 8, 1960, Macpherson recommended to the CME board that the School of Medicine be located on one campus and the campus of first choice was Loma Linda. He also recommended that the board authorize the CME administration to immediately start planning and constructing medical offices, an outpatient clinic, research laboratories, and administrative offices with a completion date of June 1964. He also recommended that the board authorize the administration to develop new organizational charts, recruit personnel, and move faculty from Los Angeles.[26]

Then suddenly the brakes were applied. Godfrey T. Anderson, president of CME; Reuben R. Figuhr, president of the General Conference; and Maynard V. Campbell, chair of the CME board of trustees, all felt that the board was not ready to decide that day. They believed that a large number of board members would vote for Los Angeles, particularly the union conference presidents. If given additional information and background, however, they would come over to the Loma Linda side.[27] Because such an important vote would need to be confirmed by the denomination's Autumn Council, the motion was officially tabled until the September board meeting.

Meanwhile, Figuhr complimented Briggs for his wholesome and beneficial influence that day: "Your last remarks near the close of the board meeting touched me deeply. We need such dedication to the cause of God as I believe has moved you to join us at the Medical School. . . . Let me say for myself that I have the fullest confidence that the Lord will lead us in the right direction. My hope of course is that it will be toward Loma Linda; yet, with all of this, our first and foremost hope must ever be that the will of the Lord be done."[28]

## The College of Medical Evangelists Becomes Loma Linda University

July 1, 1961, turned out to be a memorable day. The College of Medical Evangelists at this time had a proliferation of educational activities and diverse programs. It had become a consortium of several colleges, schools, and professional curriculums. In order to reflect these changes the name was changed to Loma Linda University (LLU).[29]

A year later Anderson proudly reported: "The sun never sets on our alumni." The number of students now totaled 1,042.[30]

Another name change signaled the school's new status. The last issue of *The Medical Evangelist* was published during the summer of 1962 and covered the first commencement of Loma Linda University. As the institution expanded into Loma Linda University, however, the administration felt that its voice and its magazine should expand its horizons. The enlarged publication—*Loma Linda University Magazine*—better reflected the institution's development.

The first issue of the *Loma Linda University Magazine* had an important news note. Certificates recognizing CME alumni as alumni of Loma Linda University were being mailed (without cost) to all alumni who had responded to an earlier invitation to receive the document. The first certificate went to Macpherson, CME's former dean, at LLU's commencement exercises, June 3, 1962. (Macpherson had just been elected to the newly created position of vice president for medical affairs at LLU.)[31]

### The Sound of Many Voices

Name changes were simple compared to the controversy over the consolidation of the Loma Linda and Los Angeles campuses in the 1960s, which seemed to continue indefinitely. The delay fostered discouragement and apathy, and made it difficult to fill faculty vacancies.[32]

The public had its own opinions. Bob Geggie, a columnist for *The Sun* newspaper, concluded that a successful consolidation in Loma Linda would "give this section of Inland Southern California the prestige of having one of the three medical schools in the Southland."[33]

Meanwhile, almost imperceptibly, staff used the term "sanitarium" less and less and the word "hospital" more and more. In fact, supported by patients now being attracted from a larger geographic area, the tendency even pointed toward developing a comprehensive "medical center."[34]

On February 8, 1960, Macpherson presented a statement to the board of trustees. It came from the full-time clinical department heads in Los Angeles. They said that in order to continue a high-quality teaching program, unification should take place *without delay.* They fully believed that the only logical, sensible, and economic move would be to consolidate in Los Angeles due to the available clinical facilities that had been developed there for almost 50 years. However, they recognized that the church leadership and the family at the Loma Linda campus did not support such a move; therefore, they recommended that the unification take place in Loma Linda as long as their conditions were met. They requested that the General Conference commit to a capital expenditure of at least $11.5 million and increase the operating budget for the school by at least $900,000.

If the General Conference could not support the first part of their proposal, then they suggested that the board vote *immediate* authorization to expand the Los Angeles campus by building a $350,000 pathology building. If a subsequent reconsideration to go to Loma Linda did *not* materialize, a gradual move to Los Angeles "would be more economical, spread the cost over a more protracted period of time and would offer much greater security as far as the School's future [was concerned]."[35] On the same day, the board appointed a consolidation committee composed of members of the board and faculty—some from each campus—to study costs, financing options, faculty recruitment, potential patients, and a proposed implementation schedule.[36]

That committee met 18 times between February 17 and September 11, 1960. On April 21 four members visited Stanford University to evaluate its recent consolidation from San Francisco to Palo Alto. Dr. Varner J. Johns, Jr., opined that, because of large financial resources for faculty recruitment and construction of facilities at Stanford University, its experience could not apply to Loma Linda. Briggs countered that the inpatient and outpatient statistics at Loma Linda for March 1960 exceeded Stanford's by 30 percent during a comparable time and that, indeed, consolidation at Loma Linda *was* feasible.[37]

### The Rainbow Book

To address the impasse, in April 1960 the board authorized the president to invite the American Medical Association and the Association of American Medical Colleges to consult with CME regarding possible consolidation. The deans of four medical colleges stepped forward.[38]

After their July 18-20, 1960, visit to both campuses, the four deans recommended unanimously that the school be consolidated in Los Angeles.[39] So, the great minds in medical education had spoken. Los Angeles should be "the place."

The board endured a paper blizzard. Faculty members of the consolidation committee from both Loma Linda and Los Angeles wheeled out the heavy artillery. They prepared information pertaining to their respective campuses. They created a "source book" for the board of trustees and the church's next Autumn Council. The committee duplicated proposals and counterproposals in different colors, leading to the designation "Rainbow Book."[40] The 82-page Rainbow Book included the 11-page report by the four deans on the liaison committee (September 7, 1960). Their conclusion read, in part, as follows:

"In reviewing all of the factors listed in the foregoing sections, the visiting committee is *of the unanimous opinion that the weight of judgment should be to consolidate on the Los Angeles Campus.* . . . The magnitude of the move to Loma Linda and the disruption in program that would occur between the time of the announced policy and the re-establishment of an effective program would present such great difficulties that we have not been able to visualize satisfactory solutions. . . . It would take at least five years to establish a program at Loma Linda once the policy decision was made, and it is not clear that in this interval the standards of the school could be maintained at an acceptable level.

"On the basis of all the information available to us and the experience personally of the several members of the visiting committee, we have been unable to recognize an alternate program of consolidation of medical education at the College of Medical Evangelists that would be reasonably certain of meeting accreditation standards. . . . The members of the visiting committee have had the opportunity of becoming familiar with the standards of medical school accreditation in the United States. In view of this we feel we would be remiss if we did not inform the Trustees and the administrative officers of the College of Medical Evangelists as well as our own Councils of our opinion. . . . We are gravely concerned that the difficulties of alternative proposals are so great that, although their possibility might be supported, their implementation is unrealistic."[41]

## Impending Disaster

Two days after this all-too-clear pronouncement, Campbell, vice president of the General Conference and chair of the CME board of trustees, wrote of a potential accreditation disaster:

"I recognize that we [the consolidation committee] are up against great odds now that the men from the Association of American Medical Colleges and the AMA have given so decided a report in favor of Los Angeles, and have made a part of their report that they see no possibility of our having a combined school at Loma Linda which could be accredited by their organization. Even before this report was given, unless the Lord intervened, it would be just a toss up which way the vote would go. However, now that we have this report, I have no doubt whatever in my mind but what both the Board and the Autumn Council will vote in favor of Los Angeles, *unless God definitely directs the minds of men.*"[42]

Expressing his faith in God, he encouraged Briggs to proceed with his part of the consolidation committee report: "It is because of the fact that I know that God is still in control and that we should not do anything to try to avoid an opportunity for Him to demonstrate His will, that I think we should go ahead with the preparation of the arguments why Loma Linda would be the better campus."[43]

## An Irresistible Force and an Immovable Object

The two sides of the Loma Linda/Los Angeles issue quickly faced off. On September 13, 1960, the CME board of trustees heard arguments in favor of consolidation in Loma Linda. The board then divided into eight groups to tour the Loma Linda campus, each led by a competent guide. The tours lasted five hours. Members then heard Briggs present a summary of reasons for consolidating in Loma Linda.[44]

The next morning the board met in Los Angeles and heard a rebuttal by Dr. Roger W. Barnes. He argued *against* the move to Loma Linda. That afternoon Briggs delivered a rebuttal to his rebuttal. In the evening Anderson asked Macpherson to give his viewpoint concerning consolidation. The latter reiterated the importance of consolidating on one campus and urged the board to decide immediately.

On the next day, however, the board remained evenly split. The chair felt that the board's recommendation to the soon-to-meet Autumn Council would carry little weight. He then posed an oddly ambiguous request to Anderson. Let the president present "an alternative plan on which the Board might come closer to unity."[45]

A flurry of activity sprang up. Anderson presented a comprehensive, 19-point, 5,050-word alternative plan. The board adopted it as Resolution #487 by a 28 to 9 vote. However, the Autumn Council, which met on November 1, 1960, did not approve the resolution. Instead they adopted a nine-point substitute resolution to be studied by the officers of the institution. Hopefully it would receive final approval at the next board meeting.[46]

Desperate for a compromise, the board actually retreated to the old two-campus model. The 1961 Autumn Council approved a September action of the board that stated that the School of Medicine would not move to either campus. Because School of Medicine authorities estimated that the last two years of the school's curriculum used less than half of the available facilities on the Los Angeles campus (including the huge Los Angeles County General Hospital) it could double the size of the school by starting a matching basic sciences program in Los Angeles. Students from the two basic sciences programs would join each other in Los Angeles during their junior year to begin clinical education.[47]

On October 25, 1961, the board voted to continue to strengthen medical education on *both* campuses of the university, with the following recommendations:

1. A four-year curriculum, including basic sciences, would be developed in Los Angeles.

2. The two-year basic sciences curriculum would be continued in Loma Linda, with those students transferring to Los Angeles for clinical experience.

3. Concurrently, the Loma Linda Division would integrate basic sciences with a to-be-developed clinical science division to establish an interdisciplinary association and collaboration between the two.

4. Then, at the time the four-year School of Medicine became operative in Los Angeles, a new two-year School of Medicine, with its own dean, would become operative in Loma Linda.[48]

## The Loma Linda Campus Grows

Seemingly in harmony with these recommendations, university administrators announced plans to increase clinical facilities in Loma Linda. The last edition of *The Medical Evangelist* announced a $4-million expansion of the hospital on the hill. Three additions were designed to acknowledge the increasingly important practice of associating clinical education facilities with basic science education. The new plans—to be built in three phases—would strengthen the emerging concept of improving clinical teaching on the Loma Linda campus.[49] It would enlarge and strengthen its staff to provide a stronger program of internships and residencies for graduates of the School of Medicine [50]

The first addition was to be a single-story, 64-bed, $600,000 psychiatric unit to be built on the east end of the hill in the shadow of the landmark water tower. (This is where the original five cottages had been built around 1900.) It would be completed in 1963. The board noted that insurance companies would pay more readily if the psychiatric unit were to be attached to the general hospital. The next year the university would build a $600,000 three-story professional building for outpatient services on the south side of the hill facing Mound Street. It would provide office space for several medical specialties, a pharmacy, outpatient X-ray facilities, and a clinical laboratory. Research laboratories would be built in the basement. This project was to start in 1964.[51]

The largest and most costly part of the enlargement, a five-story addition to the hospital, would be built at the bottom of the hill also facing south on Mound Street. It would add 75,000 square feet, and its third story would connect with the existing hospital on the hill. The $2.5-million project would include a new lobby and chapel, a teaching amphitheater and five classrooms, labor and delivery rooms, a 34-bed nursery, a volunteer's gift and snack shop, a physician's lounge and medical library, a hospital administration suite, and inpatient rooms for 88 patients. Most importantly, it would provide a completely new entrance to the Loma Linda Sanitarium and Hospital, thus relieving the congested parking on "Sanitarium Hill." A three-acre parking lot would be built across Mound Street.[52]

By December 1961 the administration had already entered negotiations with the clinical staff at Loma Linda to lease quarters in the new professional building and to decide who should practice there. In confirming a recent discussion, Anderson wrote to Dr. Raymond G. Auvil, chair of the Loma Linda Medical Group: "We are more than anxious to get moving on this building so that we can get our expanded program under way without further delay."[53]

131

Unfortunately, unanticipated difficulties arose which were of sufficient magnitude to lead to the conclusion that it was virtually impossible to implement the 1961 decision and the subsequent recommendations. Even student physicians got involved.

In May 1962 a group of 114 CME alumni, under the signature of Dr. Claude E. Steen, Sr., sent 17,000 pamphlets favoring consolidation in Loma

---

### A Defense of Loma Linda's Uniqueness
### By Brian S. Bull
#### Student physician, later dean of the School of Medicine

CME is not just another medical school. It is a school set apart—a school for the training of medical evangelists, for the educating of Christian physicians. When CME begins to fail in this respect, then it has lost its only justification for existence. . . . Time after time non-Adventists have told me why they went to a CME doctor. It was because of this something extra—this genuine feeling for and interest in humanity that CME has traditionally stamped upon its alumni.

If this something extra—"Christianity in action," if you will—is that which has ever marked CME students as a group apart, then any move toward consolidation should seriously consider whether or not the proposed unification will make it more likely that CME students will receive this mark.

There is only one way in which a student can acquire this interest in and feeling for people—that is by watching a Christian physician, backed by a loyal staff of Christian nurses, treat the whole patient. . . . This can be learned only from association with a doctor who views all patients as children of God and treats them as Jesus would have done. The only situation that meets all of these qualifications is—a Seventh-day Adventist hospital.

It was a search for this "Christianity in action" that led me to CME originally. . . . Finding this quality at CME kept me here. Hoping to be able to pass it on to future students, I have dedicated myself to teaching. For me this is CME. And should it be lost, then CME would have lost its reason for being.

It is my earnest hope that in all discussions about this problem due consideration will be given to the environment in which future medical students will get their patient contact, that CME may continue to educate medical evangelists. Very sincerely, 54

Brian S. Bull

---

Linda to members of the General Conference Committee, members of the Loma Linda University board of trustees, physicians, and ministers. These alumni, including some who helped to pioneer the school, stated that they could not stand idly by and see the school gradually lost to the church.

The alumni document referred to the decision made a year before to provide four years of medical education in Los Angeles. It also announced that a group opposed to such a move had "a will-o'-the-wisp hope." The report presented detailed arguments in opposition to consolidating in Los Angeles and the division of the school on two campuses.

A church member had written to R. R. Bietz, president of the Pacific Union Conference, complaining about CME moving to "the crowded,

### CME Alumni Argue for Loma Linda

1. Cost. Millions of dollars would need to be spent in new buildings for basic sciences.

2. Moving basic sciences to Los Angeles would weaken the school of Dentistry.

3. Because it is more difficult to recruit Seventh-day Adventist basic sciences faculty than clinical faculty, it would be more difficult for the school to avoid the teaching of evolutionary philosophy.

4. Duplication of facilities in the crime center of the leading crime city of the nation would most certainly destroy the objectives of CME and lead to the destruction of the school itself.

5. The institution was on its way to joining other religious colleges that had been secularized and were becoming "just another university."

6. It would be worse to go where God did not lead than to go alone.

7. Moving to Los Angeles would take the school from where God planted it to where He said it should never be placed.

8. Any pretense of following the "Lord's messenger" would lead to Loma Linda.

9. Moving the entire school to Loma Linda would cost far less in new buildings and operating expenses than moving to Los Angeles.

10. Loma Linda had vacant land on which to build, whereas in Los Angeles, improved property would have to be destroyed in order to build new facilities.

11. The Loma Linda campus had 510 acres, more than 20 times that of the Los Angeles campus.

12. Housing and necessary modifications to the library would cost much less in Loma Linda.

13. Construction in rural Loma Linda would cost much less than in urban Los Angeles.

14. The higher percentage of non-Adventist employees in Los Angeles, with possible involvement with labor unions, might eventually close the institution.

15. Moving everything to Los Angeles would be seen by supporting church members as a "mass violation" of the counsel given by Mrs. White with disastrous results.

16. Battle Creek became renowned throughout the world long before the Mayo Clinic was established. Had it remained true to its high calling there is every reason to believe it would still be world famous.

17. The School of Dentistry in Loma Linda had an abundance of patients, in contrast to earlier predictions. Its leaders had faith to step out on the promises of God, leaving the results with Him.

18. Leland Stanford University consolidated its entire medical college on one campus at Palo Alto and experienced an abundance of patients.[55]

wicked city of Los Angeles": "I wish it were possible for some of the members of the church to sit in on the Board meetings where we wrestle and pray and agonize over the problems facing us with the School of Medicine. . . . Certainly we need the prayers of all the believers in order to do that which God asks of His people."[56]

## The General Conference President Speaks

A few days later, Figuhr published a 10-page statement that gave a historical perspective of the debate and outlined some of the challenges in moving to Loma Linda:

1. It would weaken the clinical work of the Medical School, which was recognized as outstanding.

2. It would take a long time, if ever accomplished, to build a recognized faculty of proper standing, particularly specialists in the different fields of medicine.

3. CME would have to pay larger salaries if recognized specialists were to be recruited to Loma Linda.

4. Such a move would probably cause a loss of accreditation.

5. It would drastically reduce enrollment.

6. Such a move would disrupt already established research and clinical programs.

7. To interrupt the present program would seriously damage the church's world work.[57]

Figuhr declared that the board keenly felt their responsibility and was seeking wisdom from above. The board had been struggling with a problem that had perplexed the denomination and its leaders for nearly a quarter of a century. He also admitted that not only must a decision be made and implemented immediately, but also that such a decision would not please everybody. Regarding the upcoming verdict, he concluded, "If the decision made is right, God will bless and prosper it."[58] Figuhr urged acceptance of the board's 1961 decision:

"The board of Loma Linda University earnestly, and surely not in haste, took prayerful action to create a plan for the university that would be consistent with both the counsels of the Lord's Servant and the highest medical training standards. We believe that the plans laid can accomplish great good for the cause if we unitedly give our support to them. We invoke the cooperation of all."[59]

His comment reflected on some of the questions asked earlier by concerned members of Loma Linda's constituency: "Will our choice yield to the pressure of human logic? Or rest in faith in God? Will our decision give God opportunity to demonstrate His infinite wisdom and power?"[60]

### The Alumni Committee Speaks Again

On the other hand, the Alumni Committee published a second follow-up pamphlet in August 1962, reporting an overwhelmingly favorable response to their first one. Of hundreds of replies, only two opposed the conclusions expressed. The second brochure announced that its sponsors were proadministration. The brochure also stated that the best friends of any administration are not those who placidly acquiesce to every proposition made but are composed of those with deep convictions who have the courage to point out the dangers and pitfalls on what they see as a questionable course of action.

The document emphasized the "thousand pages of instruction from the pen of Mrs. E. G. White" regarding Loma Linda. They challenged the church paper to reprint some of her valuable instructions. Advantages outlined for providing clinical facilities in Loma Linda included:

1. A more suitable environment.
2. The mutual strengthening of education in all the schools of the university by close association with the School of Medicine.
3. The elimination of heavy operating expenses incurred by the duplication of offices, personnel, and extensive travel between the two campuses.
4. A plan that the denomination can conscientiously support, in harmony with Mrs. White's instructions.[61]

The brochure reported that the newly organized Loma Linda University board of councilors had met during the recent General Conference session in San Francisco. The group of 23 dedicated, loyal Seventh-day Adventist laymen—also successful business and professional individuals—had studied the planned expansion at the Los Angeles campus.

They expressed their conviction that centralization of the School of Medicine in Los Angeles would be an unsound financial investment. They also concluded that such a move would be detrimental to the church's youth and not be in the best interest of the denomination.

They even voted to recommend that the Loma Linda University board of trustees and members of the university's administration restudy the recent decision to enlarge facilities in Los Angeles.

When and how would the consolidation dispute ever be resolved?

---

[1] Mervyn G. Hardinge, M.D., D.Ph., Ph.D., "Consolidation of the Medical School," p. 1.

[2] Walter E. Macpherson, M.D., CME board of trustees, minutes, February 8, 1960, pp. 1-3.

[3] CME board of trustees, minutes, September 11, 1946, p. 17.

[4] *Ibid.*, September 20, 1953, p. 5.

[5] "The CME and the Los Angeles County Hospital," *CME Alumni Journal*, September 1953, p. 10; "General Hospital," *The March of CME*, (Loma Linda and Los Angeles California, the Student-Faculty Association of the College of Medical Evangelists, 1953), vol. 3, p. 59. The University of Southern California had started its second School of Medicine on September 17, 1928.

[6] Maxine Atteberry, "Something New Added, 1915 to 1924," *Pinafores to Pantsuits*, pp. 33-36.

[7] *Ibid.,* p. 37.

[8] "CME's 'Third' Campus," *The Voice of CME Employees*, March 1957, p. 3.

[9] Albert F. Brown, M.D., "Vignette of a Gentleman," *Diamond Memories*, p. 156.

[10] CME board of trustees, minutes, April 11, 1951, p. 2.

[11] *The Medical Evangelist*, November 1953, p. 6.

[12] CME board of trustees, minutes, April 9, 1953, p. 4.

[13] Francis D. Nichol, "The Location of Our Medical School," *Review and Herald*, September 17, 1953, p. 12.

[14] *The Medical Evangelist*, November 1953, pp. 6, 7.

[15] Francis D. Nichol, "What Is an Autumn Council? And How Does It Conduct Business?" *Review and Herald*, November 12, 1953, p. 10.; *The Medical Evangelist*, November 1953, pp. 6, 7; CME board of trustees, minutes, September 20, 1953, p. 4; October 22, 1953, pp. 1, 2.

[16] *The March of CME*, vol. 3, p. 89.

[17] CME board of trustees, minutes, September 11, 1958, p. 5; Glenn Calkins, January 9, 1959 letter to CME board of trustees.

[18] Council on Medical Education and Hospitals, American Medical Association, *Survey Report of College of Medical Evangelists School of Medicine*, January 6-9, 1959, included in CME board of trustees, minutes, January 28-29, 1959, p. 10.

[19] Glenn Calkins, letter to CME board of trustees, January 9, 1959. (Emphasis is in the original.) He was president of the Inter-American Division of the Seventh-day Adventist denomination and a member of the 1953 fact-finding commission at Loma Linda.

[20] Mervin G. Hardinge, M.D., Dr.Ph., Ph.D., January 23, 1959, letter to Walter P. Elliott, chair, CME board of trustees.

[21] Hardinge, "Consolidation of the Medical School," p. 2.

[22] Willis J. Hackett, November 11, 1959, letter to Bernard D. Briggs, M.D..

[23] Bernard D. Briggs, M.D., January 27, 1960, letter to Godfrey T. Anderson, Ph.D., president of CME.

[24] Ellen G. White, *Testimonies for the Church*, vol. 4, pp. 27, 28.

[25] Bernard D. Briggs, M.D., January 24, 1960, letter to Maynard V. Campbell, with copies to Reuben R. Figuhr and Godfrey T. Anderson.

[26] Walter E. Macpherson, M.D., February 8, 1960, recommendations to the CME board of trustees.

[27] Maynard V. Campbell, February 24, 1960, letter to Bernard D. Briggs, M.D.

[28] CME board of trustees, minutes, February 8, 1960, p. 2. The September board meeting would convene just before the Autumn Council.

[29] David J. Bieber, "University President Speaks at Loma Linda Convocation," *University Scope*, December 13, 1967, p. 12.

[30] Godfrey T. Anderson, Ph.D., president, "Years of Growth and Decision, Loma Linda University Quadrennial Report, 1958-1962," *Loma Linda University Magazine,* July-August 1962, p. 7.

[31] "The Latest Compendium of News, Alumni Get University Certificates," *Loma Linda University Magazine,* July-August 1962, p. 25.

[32] John E. Peterson, M.D., May 8, 1961, letter to Walter E. Macpherson, M.D.

[33] Bob Geggie, "Medical School Would Give County New Prestige," *The Sun*, August 20, 1960, p. B-1.

[34] Clarence A. Miller, "The Loma Linda San," *Diamond Memories*, pp. 24, 25.

[35] Bernard D. Briggs, "Facts and Observations Associated With the Consolidation of the School of Medicine at Loma Linda," pp. 2, 3.

[36] LLU board of trustees, minutes, February 8, 1960, p. 3.

[37] Briggs, "Facts and Observations.

[38] Liaison committee on medical education, representing the American Medical Association and the Association of American Medical Colleges, "Report of Consultation With the College of Medical Evangelists School of Medicine," July 20, 1960, p. 1. The deans were:

- W. N. Hubbard Jr., M.D., dean of the University of Michigan Medical School;
- Stanley W. Olson, M.D., dean of the Baylor University College of Medicine and member of the Executive Council of the Association of American Medical Colleges;
- William R. Willard, M.D., vice president for medical affairs and dean of the University of Kentucky College of Medicine and member of the Council on Medical Education and Hospitals of the American Medical Association;
- Thomas H. Hunter, M.D., dean of the University of Virginia School of Medicine, president of the Association of American Medical Colleges, and chair of the Executive Committee of the Association of American Medical Colleges.

[39] CME board of trustees, minutes, August 25, 1960, p. 6; CME board of trustees, "Report to the Board," August 30, 1960, p. 5.

[40] Bernard Briggs, M.D., May 25, 1993, letter to Raymond S. Moore, Ph.D.

[41] Liaison committee on medical education, representing the American Medical Association and the Association of American Medical Colleges, "Report of Consultation with the College of Medical Evangelists School of Medicine," July 20, 1960, pp. 7-11.

[42] Maynard V. Campbell, July 22, 1960, letter to Bernard D. Briggs, M.D. (Emphasis mine.)

[43] Maynard V. Campbell, July 22, 1960, letter to Bernard D. Briggs, M.D.

[44] CME board of trustees, minutes, September 13, 1960, pp. 1, 2.

[45] *Ibid.*, September 15, 1960, pp. 1, 2.

[46] *Ibid.*, November 1, 1960, pp. 1, 2.

[47] "School of Medicine to Stay on Two Campuses," *The Voice for Loma Linda University Employees*, November 1961, p. 1; Reuben R. Figuhr, "A Statement on Loma Linda University," *Review and Herald*, July 19, 1962, pp. 4-8.

[48] "Recommendation to the President and the Trustees of Loma Linda University," May 18, 1962.

[49] *The Medical Evangelist,* May-June 1962, pp. 9, 19-21.

[50] "School of Medicine to Stay on Two Campuses," *The Voice for Loma Linda University Employees,* November 1961, p. 1.

[51] "School of Medicine to Stay on Two Campuses," *The Sun,* June 1, 1962, city page. See also LLU board of trustees, minutes, January 29, 1963, p. 1.

[52] *Ibid.,* See also "Major Growth Planned for LL," *The Voice for Loma Linda University Employees,* June 1962, pp. 1, 2.

[53] Godfrey T. Anderson, December 12, 1961, letter to Raymond G. Auvil, M.D.

[54] Brian S. Bull, letter to R. R. Figuhr, president, General Conference of Seventh-day Adventists, September 8, 1960. Dr. Bull was one of the student physicians who got involved in the consolidation crisis. He was a member of the last class to graduate from CME.

[55] *The Future of Loma Linda.* Pamphlet by members of the CME Alumni, May 1962.

[56] R. R. Bietz, letter to Grace Wich, June 4, 1962.

[57] Statement by Reuben R. Figuhr, president of the General Conference, *Loma Linda University,* June 28, 1962, pp. 6, 7.

[58] Statement by Reuben R. Figuhr, president of the General Conference, *Loma Linda University,* June 28, 1962, p. 8; Reuben R. Figuhr, "Statement on Loma Linda University," *®Review and Herald,* July 19, 1962, pp. 4, 7-8.

[59] Reuben R. Figuhr, "Statement on Loma Linda University," *Review and Herald,* July 19, 1962, p. 8.

[60] "Report to the Board," CME board of trustees, minutes, August 30, 1960, pp. 18, 19.

[61] *The Future of Loma Linda*, pamphlet by members of the CME Alumni, August 1962.

# Chapter 11

# Enter Dr. David B. Hinshaw, Sr., M.D.

A mid the consolidation confusion, a young CME faculty member stepped forward. An assistant professor of surgery, Dr. David B. Hinshaw, Sr. (class of 1947) played a unique role during "the controversy of the century."

First of all, he contracted hepatitis. Then, because he was unable to work for two or three months, he decided to study the writings of Ellen White. "I read everything there was about it. What is essentially my view is that the school was established obviously on this [Loma Linda] locality. There is nothing to suggest that from the point of view of the Church at the founding of the school that it was intended to be anywhere else. Mrs. White, of course, made a statement that this would become [an important] educational center. . . . How was the Church going to walk away from here in view of that? This was a crisis involving Mrs. White's writings at the time."[1]

With the support of the younger faculty of the Department of Surgery and with a decision by the older departmental leaders, Hinshaw became chair of the Department of Surgery on July 1, 1961.[2] The appointment, of course,

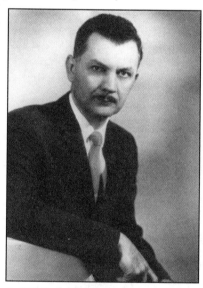

David B. Hinshaw Sr., M.D.

thrust him into the middle of the consolidation controversy. Under his leadership the department grew in stature, obtained important research grants, published its research, and presented papers in various venues.

Anderson, president of Loma Linda University, and Campbell, chair of the board of trustees, asked Hinshaw if he would become the new dean of the School of Medicine in 1962. "Things are at a real crisis, and we've got to have some leadership here, and we think you can do it."

"Sure, I'll do it," the 38-year-old doctor replied, "but I don't know that I want to do it for very long. And I'm not willing to give up the chairmanship of the Department of Surgery." So, he became dean on July 1, 1962, *and* retained his leadership of the Department of Surgery.[3]

### No Halfway Maneuver

A few months after becoming dean but before the new building plans in Loma Linda could be implemented, Hinshaw conducted informal discussions among key members of the Loma Linda faculty. How was he going to break through the barrier of indecision and delay?

"I surveyed the situation in a variety of ways, and it became quickly evident that this was an impossible situation. . . . The Loma Linda campus was rapidly disintegrating under the influence of this particular decision, and no progress had been made in creating the physical structure and faculty recruitment which would have been necessary to create a basic science unit at the Los Angeles site. . . . Very quickly it became clear that the need to revisit the question was inescapable. A firm decision had to be made one way or the other. There should be a complete consolidation on one side or the other, as opposed to some sort of halfway maneuver, which was simply unworkable."[4]

From those discussions Hinshaw determined that he would be unable to organize an Adventist preclinical faculty in Los Angeles. At the same time, with logic on their side, departmental leaders in Los Angeles sincerely felt that moving to Loma Linda would result in dissolving the school. Hundreds acting as volunteer faculty in the Los Angeles Division were not about to move to Loma Linda. Feelings were strong on both sides. As the controversy intensified, the question of consolidating the School of Medicine on one campus reemerged, full force.[5]

Out of sheer frustration, Hinshaw eventually approached Anderson with an ultimatum: "There has to be a clear-cut decision made or the School is finished. It will never survive a visit [by the accreditation survey team, slated for January 1963]. What we have to have is a firm decision and go for it whatever it's going to be. I'll support a firm decision, but I won't support this wobbling around business. That's surefire death for an institution."

Anderson called Campbell at the General Conference: "We've got to come back and talk to you." Hinshaw and Anderson flew to Washington, D.C., and in an all-day session, talked with Campbell and Figuhr. Hinshaw reiterated his position that a clear-cut decision *had* to be made.

The subsequent conversation went straight to the heart of the matter:

**Figuhr**: "Do you believe it is possible to move the School from Los Angeles to Loma Linda?"

**Hinshaw**: "Yes, I do believe it is possible. Difficult, but possible."

**Figuhr**: "What do you think is the better thing to do in the long run?"

**Hinshaw**: "I believe it is better to move it to Loma Linda for several reasons. One is we have the land. We have elbow room, space. In Los Angeles we are trapped. We would have to condemn property, and it is in a deteriorating neighborhood and a critical issue is that we will be forever deeply involved in the County Hospital."[6]

(In Hinshaw's judgment continuing with the county hospital was a huge issue—one that would marginalize Loma Linda University. He believed that dependence on the enormous city facility would compromise Loma Linda University's identity. Loma Linda needed to focus on its own university hospital where it would have its own separate identity.)

**Figuhr**: "If the board votes to move it out to Loma Linda, can you do it?"

**Hinshaw**: "I believe it can be done if the Church gets behind it, and I believe it's the right thing to do."

**Figuhr**: "Let's do it!"

He and Campbell then immediately began to discuss the importance of the next board meeting, which was coming up in September. They had committed themselves to move to Loma Linda.[7] In anticipation of the crucial board meeting, Steen wrote to fellow alumni requesting that they send special delivery letters to each board member urging a firm and kind, but positive stand on consolidation in Loma Linda.

The September 1962 board meeting met at the White Memorial Hospital to address the consolidation issue once and for all. Hinshaw declared that as dean he would support whatever the board decided, but that his own preference was that the school should move to Loma Linda. Figuhr then made it clear that the board should vote to consolidate in Loma Linda: "The Dean has said it is possible to do."[8]

Dr. Keld Reynolds commented: "The young Dean generated a sort of infectious courage which led the Board to hope that this David just might have the right stone for felling the 'Goliath of Indecision.'"[9]

### They Did It!

On September 25, 1962, with escalating concern from university alumni and church leaders favoring Loma Linda, the board voted with *a solid majority* to consolidate the two campuses in Loma Linda. Another motivation was the increasingly difficult but seldom publicly mentioned political realities at the Los Angeles County General Hospital. Still, there would be many more rivers to cross before this momentous action could become a reality.

The Loma Linda University board of trustees minutes reveal that Hinshaw not only sought direction from the board but that he also asked for explicit, unambiguous authority to implement the decision they would make that day:

Anderson presented Hinshaw as dean of the School of Medicine, and indicated that Hinshaw wished to discuss with the board membership what his duties were to be and how he was to relate himself to future plans for the School of Medicine. Hinshaw indicated that he had great need of more clarification from the board of trustees concerning the future development of the School of Medicine, if he were to efficiently carry out his work as dean of the school. He presented to the trustees a number of alternative ways by which the School of Medicine could develop. He declared positively that he made no recommendation of any one plan. He was ready to serve under any of them.

In his presentation Hinshaw emphasized the need to establish *one* primary base and not to be under the heavy cost of developing two main bases.

As usual, one committee spawned another, and the committee that was appointed by the officers the previous day prepared and brought into the next meeting a plan for development in Loma Linda. The board gave general approval to the suggested plan, but appointed yet another subcommittee to restudy it and bring in a more clearly defined plan.

During the same meetings, the board took a second vote. These few words emphasize the most important points in the decision, simplify the wording, and illustrate the intensity of feelings that brought the controversial action to a vote. "Some of the Trustees felt that it would be well to declare in emphatic form re-emphasizing the decision to develop the School of Medicine on the Loma Linda campus as in Action #1017 above." Then, under Action #1032, we read: "Voted that the four-year program of the School of Medicine be developed on the Loma Linda campus of the Loma Linda University, in effect continuing the teaching of the basic sciences on that campus and transferring to the Loma Linda campus the junior and senior classes as soon as clinical facilities can be made available."[10]

These decisions gave Hinshaw approval to assume the unequivocal authority he would need to implement the board's decision. Now it became necessary to greatly expand the Loma Linda facilities for the School of Medicine and the School of Nursing.

Also, a new university hospital/teaching/research facility (the 516-bed Loma Linda University Hospital) was about to be born.

### Why Was Loma Linda Chosen?

That night after the board meeting Hinshaw and Campbell met with the medical staff to explain what had happened. Some asked, "Is there something we can do to reverse this?"

"No."

"Well, why not?"

Discussion was fruitless. Eventually, Hinshaw and Campbell simply closed down the meeting.[11]

Hinshaw defended the reasons for the Loma Linda choice: "The institution possessed sufficient real estate on the Loma Linda site to provide for long-term development. In addition, it was felt that this course of action would be much more acceptable to the sponsoring church body at large. It would also be more consistent with the perceived destiny of Loma Linda as it was originally envisioned at the time the institution was founded."[12]

Figuhr assessed these historic developments and set forth his views: "It goes without saying that boards rarely take actions that please everyone. The action of a year ago did not please all. It is too much to expect that the present one will. But boards must act upon the best information available. It happens sometimes that after a board has taken an action, conditions change and more facts are brought to light. When this happens, a wise board reconsiders. It would be irrational to do otherwise. A year ago certain facts and information were not available that have come to light since. This is what led the board of the Loma Linda University to reconsider its action of a year ago.

"It is the earnest hope that now, at last, after many years of fervent discussion and long hours of study, the question of the location of the four years of medical training has been settled. Efforts to move in other directions appear to have proved impractical. Indications are that this seems to be the way the Lord wants us to move. Let us all face with faith and courage the uncertainties, the risks, and the problems, confident that God is with us."[13]

## Calming the Storm

Hinshaw called his first faculty meeting in early November 1962. He felt some anxiety because it included more than just the medical staff. The Thomason Amphitheater at the White Memorial Hospital was packed for the occasion. Following prayer and a few preliminary statements, a preeminent, influential senior surgeon asked for the floor. "I want to make a motion," he announced, "that this body take an action to send a letter from the faculty to the Accrediting Council for Medical Schools recommending that they put the School on immediate probation until the Board meets and rescinds this ridiculous action."

Recalling the event years later, Hinshaw said, "Well, that put a little spice in the evening to get started. I was being tested." The board was gone, and there wasn't a sympathetic eye in the audience except for a few people who had slipped in from Loma Linda. The motion was met with cheers, practically a standing ovation. In response, Hinshaw said, "With all due respect, your motion is out of order and unacceptable, Number One. Number Two, this meeting is adjourned. I will call another faculty meeting when I see fit."

He then left and didn't call another faculty meeting for two years. Hinshaw did what he perceived had to be done. Acknowledging that he had become a polarizing figure, he said, "So, you see where my reputation came of being a tough, miserable so-and-so, who won't listen to anybody, just as mean as sin and tough as nails and iron. But that became useful to me. I had to be that for a while. I did realize that there was no way I could get anything done by constructing some kind of committee. I couldn't get a committee together on any subject that would support what had to be done. Everybody thought this was the end of the School. Obviously, I had lost my mind or been seduced or something."[14]

## Ironing Out the Wrinkles

Dr. John E. Peterson, Sr. (class of 1939), associate dean and former chair of the Department of Medicine, favored the move to Loma Linda and became very helpful during the transition. "The institution owes him a lot," Hinshaw reflected.

When the two had consultations, several issues quickly became evident. The "Hospital on the Hill" was hopelessly inadequate, and a new medical center had to be built. The school would also have to develop hospital affiliations in the area. On top of it all, its leaders would have to stabilize relationships with the Los Angeles County General Hospital until they could move students to Loma Linda.

For a number of months Hinshaw had no assurance that any of the clinical faculty in Los Angeles would move to Loma Linda. He conducted passionate, soul-searching meetings in people's homes and in restaurants. A small group of faculty members started planning the new medical center. Circumstances and time constraints required Hinshaw to continue to conduct a reasonably benevolent dictatorship. "I did a lot of arbitrary things," he acknowledged. "We made decisions rapidly. We had to."

Once the shock was over, faculty members began responding to inquiries regarding their needs for the upcoming move to Loma Linda, which would occur in stages. Hinshaw also recruited some of the younger graduates who were more receptive to the forthcoming move than their elders.

Meanwhile, Hinshaw maintained an affiliation for juniors at the Los Angeles County General Hospital. He also developed a mutually beneficial affiliation with Riverside County General Hospital. The hospital in Loma Linda was somewhat helpful in providing clinical experience. Hinshaw also established a pediatrics program for seniors at the large hospital at nearby March Air Force Base.

As new members of the faculty arrived, "People started to come out of the woodwork," Hinshaw said. "and [a new clinical faculty] took shape." It had to be a fresh start. In time, most of the tensions dissipated. Although Hinshaw went to both campuses for a while, he gradually moved the dean's office to Loma Linda.

In November 1962 Hinshaw delivered a progress report to the board on the development of long-range plans. He stressed the need of maintaining the *status quo* so that no deterioration in teaching would occur. He reported that recruitment of clinical faculty for the Loma Linda campus did not seem to be a problem. Also, he had developed an understanding with the University of Southern California to assume responsibilities resulting from any decrease in activity by Loma Linda University at the Los Angeles County General Hospital.[15]

## Accreditation Challenges

As Hinshaw prepared for the upcoming January 1963 accreditation survey, the controversy intensified. "All we could do for the visit was plan as well as we could and pray that the Lord would send us the right people and contacts who would understand the circumstances," he said. The survey went well at the beginning, with the team spending two days in Los Angeles and two days in Loma Linda. Some members were extremely helpful, but the secretary of the group was quite antagonistic.

In the midst of the visit, the secretary dropped and broke his thick glasses. He became virtually helpless. Peterson acquired lens prescriptions over the phone and had a new pair of glasses for him within 24 hours. Diplomacy dissipated the tense atmosphere, and the man was extremely grateful.

Hinshaw took the team to Peterson's home at the top of Lawton Avenue for a panoramic view of the San Bernardino Valley. The weather was perfect—the January sky was brilliant, and the mountains beautiful. The team had come from Chicago and Pittsburgh where it had been raining and snowing for a considerable time. Hinshaw pointed to an orange grove and said,

"That's where the new Medical Center will be built, and it will be built for you men to see the next time you come."[16]

In spite of obvious conflict, the team judged that the students were being adequately served. In the end, they had to congratulate the institution on making a clear-cut decision. Although they recognized that there were many difficulties to overcome, they gave Hinshaw and his team an A for enthusiasm. They recognized that a young faculty team had a good chance of making the consolidation work. They also recognized that the Seventh-day Adventist Church strongly supported the move, so they recommended continued full accreditation. As soon as the teaching program had fully materialized on the Loma Linda campus, they promised to be back. In the meantime, they called for a progress letter once a year.

"Well, you couldn't ask for more than that," Hinshaw concluded. "They left, and people in the city [of Los Angeles] were horrified. How could we have conned this informed group of people?"[17]

In the meantime the formerly antagonistic secretary's supervisor on the liaison committee on medical education didn't like the conclusions on the survey. He summoned Hinshaw to Chicago. "You young whippersnapper," he chided. "You're not dry behind the ears. What do you think you're doing messing around with things like this?" He gave Hinshaw a good stiff lecture about the fact that it was obvious he didn't know what he was getting into. Hinshaw let the man talk until he finally got tired and quit. But the man still wanted to talk with the head of Hinshaw's church.

Hinshaw arranged for him to meet Board Chair Campbell and General Conference President Figuhr. As soon as they reached the supervisor's office, he started lecturing the church leaders. In addition to the fact that in his opinion the men didn't know what they were getting into, he didn't believe in church-related institutions of higher education anyway. He vowed he would never set foot on their campus because he just couldn't stand it. "I don't want to have anything to do with it," he said.

He wanted Figuhr to understand that the venture would cost a lot of money and wondered if the church backed the project. He looked at Figuhr, pointed at Hinshaw, and asked, "Are you backing him or aren't you?"

A steady man, Figuhr took it all in calmly: "Well doctor, we appreciate your counsel and remarks, and I am sure there is much wisdom in what you say, but we want you to know that we are firmly behind the Dean here and the Church will see to it that the resources are available."

The man said, "Well, all right, I don't know what you're getting into, but all right. All right, if you *must*."

According to Hinshaw, Figuhr then received an incredible number of complaints about the matter. Knowing that major developments needed time to mature, however, he would quietly respond by saying, "I'll look into it"; "If there's anything to this, I'll get back to you"; "Have patience"; or "We believe the Lord is going with us in this."[18]

From the beginning, Hinshaw believed the consolidation of the School of Medicine in Loma Linda would eventually succeed or he would not have attempted it. From the 1967 site visit forward he knew it would work. He acknowledges that the institution was "sailing in choppy waters, but there was no risk of being swamped."

Because the new hospital had no patients, the accreditation team decided to send a small group back in three years. When they returned in 1970, the hospital was packed with patients!

## Now What About White Memorial Hospital?

The board spent a considerable amount of time discussing what to do with the White Memorial Hospital. Back on August 27, 1963, it appointed a representative committee of 15 individuals to develop a comprehensive plan for the future role of the hospital. Because the committee desired further direction, a special meeting of the board was called in Dayton, Ohio, where many of the board members attended a meeting of conference presidents. With broad guidelines, the committee was to begin deliberations in October.[19]

Less than a month later, board members decided to arrange for the hospital to be operated either by the Pacific Union Conference or the Southern California Conference, recognizing the probable need to finance improvements from long-term borrowed capital.[20] The board then voted to adopt recommendations submitted by the special committee to transfer ownership of the $7.5-million facility[21] to the Southern California Conference. They made a few suggestions for the move:

1. That the transfer be based on a 50-year lease—as soon as possible—and not later than December 31, 1963.

2. That accounts receivable and accounts payable be negotiated by an appropriate committee.

3. That all personnel housing, furniture, and hospital equipment be transferred, except some research equipment not needed for hospital use.

4. That Loma Linda University retain the right to continue operating various schools within the White Memorial Hospital on terms to be negotiated.[22]

Although the staff at the White Memorial Hospital at first felt betrayed, in time almost everyone recognized the advantages to both institutions and to the denomination. The board then voted to recommend affiliation agreements covering residency training programs and undergraduate programs in nursing, dietetics, medical technology, and radiologic technology. They would base these affiliations on detailed contracts written by joint committees, approved by the respective boards, and subject to university policy and the agreement of the General Conference.[23]

Library books would be transferred to Loma Linda, with the exception of duplicates. These could become the basis for a medical library for interns and residents at the White Memorial Hospital.[24] The General Conference Placement Service would move to Loma Linda as soon as possible.[25]

## Other Innovations

Several decisions had to be made at this point. They illustrated the many complexities of consolidation. The "shopping list" was a long one:

1. A new nonprofit corporation had to be established at the White Memorial Hospital.

2. Donors for the proposed library needed to be notified.

3. The Personnel Department had to be divided.

4. Departmental leadership had to be clarified.

5. Insurance policies for buildings, equipment, and employee health had to be rewritten.

6. Rental agreements for housing for nursing and dietetic students, including utilities and maintenance, had to be arranged.

7. The Credit Department had to be split.

8. Remaining university offices needed to be consolidated.

9. Inventories needed to be taken.

10. Contracts for radiology and pathology needed to be renegotiated.

11. An interim, five-member advisory board of management would (diplomatically) represent both the university and the conference until a new board of trustees could be formed (December 31, 1963). They would operate the hospital and clinic, coordinate adjustments, and take care of any complications.[26]

On July 1, 1964, the board voted to phase out the undergraduate students' participation in the outpatient clinics, except for pediatrics and OB/GYN, which were subject to minor adjustments. The board joined the Southern California Conference in requesting the General Conference to authorize a loan of up to $3 million for improvements, working capital, housing needs, etc., in Los Angeles.[27]

Tor Lidar, managing editor of *University Scope*, anticipated questions from the Loma Linda community and solicited opinions from local citizens. The Loma Linda Chamber of Commerce quoted County of San Bernardino planners as forecasting that Loma Linda's population would triple to "a whopping 17,000" in a few years. Lidar reported that both churches on campus, as well as the Loma Linda Academy and elementary school, were ready to expand their plants to meet the projected growth. Beginning in the fall of 1963, both churches would conduct two church services, one at 8:15 a.m. and one at 11 a.m. Hospital administrator Clarence A. Miller projected that the membership of the faculty, student body, and churches would more than double.[28]

Postmaster Olsen O. Wheeler said that the Loma Linda population numbered almost 6,000 and that the post office could handle four to five times that many people. Real Estate Broker Clarence R. Appleton reported that 200 acres had been earmarked for new homes and apartments. Some low-cost housing would be in the range of $11,000 to $12,000, with others priced as high as $30,000. The E. J. Miller Construction Company had already started subdividing several tracts near the university.

The community was preparing for the expected growth and so was the university. The size of the library stacks had doubled, but additional space would be needed for acquisition, processing, and cataloguing departments. The new university-owned supermarket had developed a strong business since its recent relocation. It was in a position to triple its clientele. The Campus Pharmacy would conclude its remodeling with a new bookstore by September 16, 1963.[29]

## Hinshaw Interview on Consolidation

Q: "Doctor Hinshaw, do you have any answer for your critics who have charged that you do make sweeping changes and decisions without consulting them?"

A: "The Dean of a School of Medicine does not seek popularity. Certain decisions must be made whether or not they please everybody. Certain executive decisions have to be made by the Dean of the School of Medicine. My primary concern must be with the School."

Q: "Reportedly a large number of faculty members in Los Angeles are leaving us for positions on the faculty of neighboring Medical Schools, primarily USC and the California College of Medicine. Is there any truth to this?"

A: "Quite naturally there are many competent faculty members in the Los Angeles area whose practice and social interests hold them there, who have been sought as faculty members by other schools in the Los Angeles area, and we are pleased to help these teachers make a transfer under these circumstances; however, there has been no general exodus of faculty members."

Q: "Do you consider the affiliation with the Riverside County Hospital a success?"

A: "I do. Although this obviously is in an early stage, it has gone along with remarkable smoothness, and the administrative personnel at the hospital and in the County as well as the attending staff and physicians in Riverside have given splendid cooperation and support to the program."

Q: "How does this affiliation work? What is the arrangement between Loma Linda University and the Riverside County Hospital?"

A: "An affiliation agreement between the University and the County Board of Supervisors has been developed and signed. This provides for mutual interchange and benefit between the two organizations."

Q: "Has a name been settled upon for the new complex here in Loma Linda?"

A: "To my knowledge no name has been settled upon, but I presume it will be the Loma Linda University Medical Center."

Q: "How soon will faculty members from Los Angeles and other areas move to Loma Linda to take up teaching responsibilities?"

A: "Some faculty members have already moved all or part of their activities to Loma Linda."

Q: "At the present time the junior class of medicine receives virtually all of its training at the Los Angeles County [General] Hospital and the senior class is traditionally educated at the White Memorial Hospital. Assuming that it takes four years for us to complete the Medical Center at Loma Linda, and assuming further that between now and the completion of the facilities at Loma Linda it should become necessary to move out the medical students who are now at the White Memorial Hospital, are there adequate educational facilities into which these students could be placed and not be interrupted in their education?

A: "Yes, indeed! The Medical School has perfectly adequate affiliations in other hospitals with which to carry on the full student teaching program."[30]

Jerry L. Pettis, vice president for public relations and development and editor-in-chief of the *University Scope*, conducted a hardball interview with Hinshaw regarding the consolidation.[31] Earlier he had editorialized his intention for the weekly campus newspaper:

"This seems a good time to put in the record what we stand for. We will countenance no editorial bias, there will be no secrets, and we will endeavor to present all sides of serious questions facing the Administration or Trustees. . . .

"In other words, we will do our best to tell the whole story. Maybe we are naïve, but somehow we believe that if the people have ALL the facts, then truth, equity and justice will prevail."[32]

**Managing People**

Hinshaw conducted few faculty meetings during those volatile years. He did, however, schedule a major retreat in Santa Barbara over one weekend. He wanted to recruit people who conceivably could work together. He invited them to be part of something wonderful and great. People met in small groups, laid some plans, and tried to work through issues. It got people to thinking about new curricula.[33]

In 1991, after Hinshaw had become president of Loma Linda University Medical Center, he was asked, "How did the Medical School's accrediting body react to its consolidation at Loma Linda?" This was a vital question, considering that the AMA had unanimously voted in favor of Los Angeles:

"The accreditation of the Medical School during these years was always firm and was never under question. The Medical School class size was modestly reduced for several years during the early years of consolidation of the medical program. It was quickly brought back, however, to its previous size and eventually was increased.

"A number of key faculty members in the clinical area were moved from Los Angeles to Loma Linda, but a large recruiting effort was made to bring in new individuals as well. As would be natural, a high percentage of those who moved from the Los Angeles site were among the younger elements of the faculty. This group was a very dedicated, hard-working, vibrant team, and have been key in the development of the institution."[34]

The hotly debated issue of "clinical training" has long since been resolved. Today, students in the various schools of the university acquire clinical experience at Loma Linda University Medical Center, as well as its Children's Hospital, East Campus Hospital, Rehabilitation Institute, Heart and Surgical Hospital, and Behavioral Medicine Center. In addition they obtain clinical experience at Riverside County Regional Medical Center, Arrowhead Regional Medical Center (the San Bernardino County Hospital), the Jerry L. Pettis Memorial Veterans Medical Center, Kaiser Permanente (both Fontana and Riverside), the Betty Ford Hospital in Palm Desert, and in Los Angeles at the White Memorial Medical Center and Glendale Adventist Medical Center.

The university also maintains affiliations with the Hinsdale Hospital near Chicago, the Kettering Medical Center in Ohio, Florida Hospital in Orlando, and health-professional offices scattered throughout the United States. Students for International Mission Service (SIMS) cares for the underserved at clinics and hospitals around the world.

### White Memorial Hospital Is Formally Adopted

In October 1963 the Loma Linda University board of trustees, meeting at the denomination's Autumn Council in Washington, D.C., transferred ownership of the $7.5-million, 308-bed, White Memorial Hospital and Clinic to the Southern California Conference of Seventh-day Adventists, effective January 1, 1964. The action also called for a plan of affiliation between the two institutions.[35]

### Comments on Consolidation

Cree Sandefur, president of the Southern California Conference, said that

## UNIVERSITY HOSTS AMA PRESIDENT
(An editorial by Jerry L. Pettis, vice president for public relations and development)

Mrs. Pettis and I had the pleasure last weekend of having as our guest Dr. Edward R. Annis, President of the American Medical Association and President-elect of the World Medical Association. During his stay in southern California, Dr. Annis visited the Loma Linda University campus. He met with teachers and students and saw plans for the School of Medicine's consolidation at Loma Linda.

As we drove back to the airport for our flight to Los Angeles, he made some comments which I would like to pass on editorially:

This is a nice location. I'd like to be a medical student in an atmosphere like this. . . . Loma Linda University students should be greatly inspired by those who have gone before them, serving their country and their church in such exemplary and humanitarian fashion throughout the world.

I like the design for your new Loma Linda [University] Medical Center. It is one of the best plans I've seen. . . . One of the most inspiring experiences I've had since becoming an officer of the AMA was a meeting with members of the National Association of Seventh-day Adventist Dentists several months ago in Florida. These men were more than well-trained dentists—they were professional people with a significant purpose in life . . . and to my mind, this joy of living and commitment to humanitarian goals is best inculcated by religiously oriented universities. . . . Your graduates serving primitive peoples unselfishly in many lands comprised a peace corps long before the idea gained political popularity.

I hope I may come back when your physical plant is completed. I like what you are setting about to do here.

This sort of spontaneous enthusiasm for our program and objectives encourages me. It reminds me of the many nice things Vice-president Lyndon Johnson said when he visited the West Coast recently. Our University does have a great past and, in my book, it has an even greater future. I'd far rather share the optimism of such than join the "crepe hangers" who find the challenge of change and growth disturbing.

Loma Linda University is a great institution with a wonderful mission. Give it a little faith, love and confidence and a lot of hard work and it will be even greater. What do you think? JLP[36] the affiliation would add strength to the excellence of patient care at the White Memorial Hospital and to the educational opportunities at the university. The clinical training for School of Medicine seniors would continue at the White Memorial Hospital until phased out. He emphasized that both the university and the hospital were part of the Seventh-day Adventist Church and that the transfer would not in any way disrupt the hospital's health services to the public.[37]

The initial response to the change of ownership at the hospital seemed to be positive. Pettis wrote a cheerful editorial in the *University Scope*:

"During the past week we have had a delightful experience. From conversations with employees, medical students, interns, residents and physician staff members at the White Memorial Hospital we have come to a satisfying conclusion. The prospect of transferring this Medical Center to the Southern California Conference for the love, affection and local management to which it is entitled has brought about an enthusiastic response in every quarter.

"To everyone the proposal of the Loma Linda University Trustees to have 'the White' operated by a Los Angeles oriented and 'based' hospital Board makes sense and assures this well known and highly respected hospital a continuing prominent place in the family of Seventh-day Adventist medical institutions.

"From the maintenance department to the Administrator's office there is a sigh of relief and an air of expectancy. Even though all of the details haven't been worked out, enough is known to give everyone a boost in morale.

"As one employee put it: 'I've worked here for ten years and this is the best news yet! I wouldn't trade it for a pay raise.'" JLP.[38]

Lidar, managing editor of the *University Scope,* reported similar responses: "The hospital and clinic staff, from chiefs of staff to messengers, have expressed approval of a change that will maintain the University affiliation although the University will no longer operate the institution. . . . It also appears that the apprehension found among some of the employees . . . was based on a feeling of uncertainty."[39]

Dr. Clarence E. Stafford, professor of surgery, described the acceptance of the agreement among his colleagues: "The change, as far as I am able to tell, is well accepted by the physicians. . . . This arrangement will make it possible to render good service and at the same time make it possible to carry on a strong intern-resident-teaching program under the affiliation with the University."[40]

Campbell, chair of the board of trustees, felt that the consolidation was the greatest challenge in the history of the institution. Over the decades, many leaders have realized that when challenges have been met, God gets the credit: "This problem has faced the school for nearly half a century, and became more acute as the years passed by. . . . However, we know that God is in control, and I am confident that He led the Trustees in taking their clear-cut and far-reaching decision." He then reported that the great majority of the alumni with whom he had had personal contact could be described as enthusiastic over the whole program.[41]

The Southern California Conference moved quickly to appoint Irwin J. Remboldt, a former administrator of the White Memorial Hospital, to become its new administrator. Remboldt was not only eminently qualified, but he had valuable experience. He would oversee the Glendale and White hospitals, which combined had more than 600 beds and a workforce of 1,700 employees.[42]

Outside of Los Angeles, Riverside County General Hospital expressed a genuine interest in the consolidation by cooperating with Loma Linda University in providing clinical experience for its students. It not only welcomed the opportunity of upgrading its medical care by becoming a teaching hospital, but it also offered facilities beyond those called for in signed contracts. It offered to build research facilities for the university's use and performed considerable remodeling to accommodate Loma Linda University students. Faculty members of the School of Medicine were happy, and student physicians felt they were receiving excellent clinical experience.[43]

In 1966 the 450-bed Riverside County General Hospital adopted a new name that displayed its affiliation with Loma Linda University—Riverside General Hospital and University Medical Center. The County of Riverside board of supervisors changed the name in response to a request by the hospital's medical staff and administration.[44]

The many years of controversy officially ended on January 2, 1964, when Loma Linda University presented the deed for the White Memorial Hospital and Clinic to the Southern California Conference. It then became the White Memorial Medical Center. Anderson, president of Loma Linda University, explained: "As we arrive at the time of making the actual transfer, we extend to the Southern California Conference our wishes for success. We don't feel that we are leaving the 'White.' Through a clinical training affiliation we will continue to have an interest in this medical center." Anderson then pledged to assist in advancing the humanitarian objectives of the White Memorial Medical Center.[45]

## Loma Linda Moves Into High Gear

In addition to the activity of local developers, Loma Linda University subdivided an orange grove into 59 lots for new members of the staff and those moving from Los Angeles. The properties varied in size from 9,000 square feet to half an acre.[46]

Architects Heitschmidt and Thomas, as well as the Ellerby Company, consulting architects from St. Paul, Minnesota, met with university officials (including Hinshaw) for five days starting on September 23, 1963. They announced that working drawings of the new university hospital could be started by the end of the year. Miller announced that the architects would "convert stated requirements into specific plans," and that the plans would be presented again to department heads at a meeting later in the year.[47]

---

[1] Merlin D. Burt and Petre Cimpoeru, oral history with David B. Hinshaw, Sr., M.D., July 16, 1996.

[2] July 1961 was the same month that the "College of Medical Evangelists" became "Loma Linda University."

[3] Burt and Cimpoeru.

[4] David B. Hinshaw Sr., M.D., "Q & A With the Presidents, David B. Hinshaw, Sr., M.D.," *Scope*, January–March 1991, p. 47.

[5] Burt and Cimpoeru.

[6] *Ibid.*

[7] *Ibid.*

[8] *Ibid.*

[9] Keld J. Reynolds, Ph.D., "If They Held Together, They Would Continue Strong," *From Vision to Reality, 1905-1980*, p. 156.

[10] LLU board of trustees, minutes, September 25-26, 1962, p. 9. Appearing here as recorded in the official board's second vote under the subtitle "School of Medicine to Go to Loma Linda Campus."

[11] Burt and Cimpoeru, op. cit.

[12] Hinshaw.

[13] Reuben R. Figuhr, "Further Statement on Loma Linda University," *Review and Herald*, October 18, 1962, pp. 16, 24.

[14] Burt and Cimpoeru.

[15] LLU board of trustees, minutes, November 27, 1962, pp. 2, 3.

[16] *Ibid.*

[17] Burt and Cimpoeru.

[18] *Ibid.*

[19] LLU board of trustees, minutes, August 27, 1963, p. 10; *Ibid.*

[20] *Ibid.*, September 20, 1963, pp. 3-5; *Ibid*, September 27, 1963, p. 1.

[21] Richard Utt, "If They Held Together, They Would Continue Strong," *From Vision to Reality, 1905-1980* (Loma Linda, California: Loma Linda University Press, 1980), p. 156.

[22] LLU board of trustees, minutes, September 20, 1963, pp. 4, 5, 9.

[23] *Ibid.*, October 20, 1963, p. 4.

[24] *Ibid.*, pp. 4, 5; "Library Books to be Transferred to LL," *University Scope*, October 25, 1963, p. 6.

[25] *Ibid.*, p. 7.

[26] *Ibid.*, pp. 4-11.

[27] *Ibid.*, pp. 11, 12.

[28] Tor Lidar, "Focus on Loma Linda Growth," *University Scope*, September 3, 1963, p. 3.

[29] *Ibid.*

[30] David B. Hinshaw, M.D., quoted by Jerry L. Pettis, "Consolidation: Theme of Dean Hinshaw Interview," *University Scope*, October 3, 1963, pp. 4, 5. Mr. Pettis eventually became the first Seventh-day Adventist to become a United States congressman, and Dean Hinshaw directed the Department of Surgery at the new 548-bed Jerry L. Pettis Memorial Veterans Medical Center that opened 14 years later in Loma Linda.

[31] Jerry L. Pettis, "Consolidation: Theme of Dean Hinshaw Interview," *University Scope*, October 3, 1963, pp. 4, 5.

[32] Jerry L. Pettis, editorial, *University Scope*, September 17, 1963, p. 2.

[33] Burt and Cimpoeru.

[34] Hinshaw, "Q & A With the Presidents," pp. 48, 49.

[35] "Trustees Finalize SC Conference Ownership of 'White Memorial,'" *University Scope,* October 25, 1963, p. 1.

[36] Jerry L. Pettis, "University Hosts AMA Pres.," *University Scope*, September 27, 1963, p. 2.

[37] "Trustees Finalize SC Conference Ownership"

[38] Jerry L. Pettis, "Best News Yet," *University Scope*, October 18, 1963, p. 2.

[39] Tor Lidar, "Smog of Apprehension Clears as News of Conference Reins Reaches 'White,'" *University Scope*, November 1, 1963, p. 4.

[40] *Ibid.*

[41] Maynard V. Campbell, "Chairman of Trustees Outlines Loma Linda University Growth," *University Scope,* December 6, 1963, p. 4.

[42] "Remboldt Named General Administrator for White Memorial, Glendale Hospitals," *University Scope*, December 6, 1963, p. 5. Remboldt not only administered the nearby Glendale Sanitarium and Hospital, but also was a member of the Loma Linda University board of trustees, the American College of Hospital Administrators, the Hospital Council of Southern California board of directors, and the Executive Committee of the General Conference of Seventh-day Adventists.

[43] Maynard V. Campbell, "Chairman of Trustees Outlines Loma Linda University Growth," *University Scope*, December 6, 1963, p. 4.

[44] "Riverside Hospital Adds 'University' to Official Title," *University Scope*, May 6, 1966, p. 1.

[45] Godfrey T. Anderson, Ph.D., "WMH Deed Presented to SC Conference," *University Scope*, January 3, 1964, p. 6.

[46] "University to Subdivide 59 Lots for LA and New Staff Members," *University Scope*, December 6, 1963, p. 5.

[47] "Architects Expect Working Drawings on Medical Center to Begin in 1964," *University Scope*, October 3, 1963, p. 1.

# Chapter 12:

# Loma Linda
# University Medical Center

T he preliminary plans for the new university hospital in Loma Linda were well advanced by January 31, 1964. In fact they were finalized enough to project 1967 as a completion date. According to Robert L. Cone,

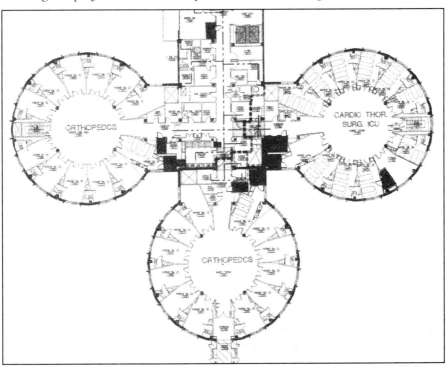

Although other hospitals had used the shape, this would become the first university hospital to be built with the cloverleaf design.[1] A wedge-shaped bathroom separated each patient room.

TGV1-6

vice president for financial affairs and chair of the planning committee, students entering professional curricula at the university in the fall of 1967 would be the first to complete their education within the new facility.[2]

The nine-story, 320-bed hospital with twelve operating rooms would be built on a 20-acre plot south of the University church. Plans showed three circular, five-story towers, which would be built in a cloverleaf formation. Offices, outpatient facilities, and support services were to be located in the "stem" of the cloverleaf.[3]

Ground-breaking ceremonies for the new medical center in Loma Linda convened on commencement weekend, June 7, 1964. Witnessed by 1,200 people, including local city and county politicians, the one-hour event featured university officers and Figuhr, president of the General Conference, speaking on "Fulfilling Our World Mission." Dr. Dwight L. Wilbur, editor of *California Medicine* and clinical professor of medicine at Stanford University School of Medicine, presented a speech titled "The Challenge of Modern Medical Education."[4]

### The Contractors

As a joint venture, contractors Larry C. Havstad and Associates and the

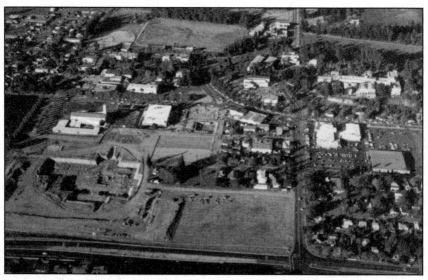

Arial view of the building site.

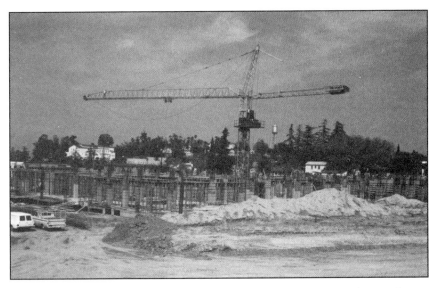

The massive, half-million-square-foot,[5] concrete-and-steel structure began to emerge. The controversial vote to consolidate the School of Medicine in Loma Linda now—at last—began to meet with increasing approval.

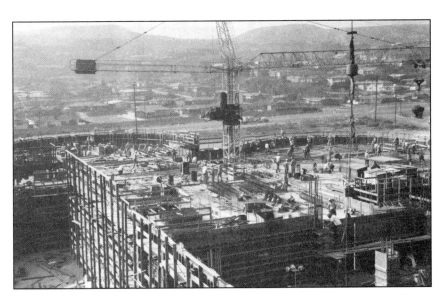

The new Loma Linda University Medical Center consisted of four structures, separated by seismic joints. The buildings could move independently during an earthquake. One hundred subcontractors, with as many as 700 workmen, "fast-tracked" the new hospital in less than three years.[6]

Del E. Webb Corporation began excavations on August 19. The Heitschmidt-Havstad team had become famous for stretching the CME/LLU building dollar. Havstad had already erected an astonishing number of buildings for the Seventh-day Adventist Church.[7]

His architect for almost 40 years, Earl T. Heitschmidt, joined Havstad in adapting to the financial constraints that faced the institution. Together they saved millions of dollars. On occasion, Havstad personally absorbed costs that normally would be charged to the owners. Because of Havstad, Webb, and Heitschmidt's combined efforts, the total cost for building and equipping the new university hospital was more than $10 million less than the $33 million originally estimated.[8]

As construction proceeded, Dean Hinshaw anticipated future growth. He persuaded the board of trustees to enlarge the new hospital's three circular, five-story towers to seven stories. On May 25, 1965, the board authorized construction of the two additional stories, acknowledging that the cost would increase considerably if delayed until a later time. The additional space would increase the hospital's bed capacity from 320 to 516. The board also added a sixth floor to the outpatient wing to accommodate the School of Nursing.[9]

### The Clinical Faculty at LLU

Hinshaw then successfully convinced several dozen clinical faculty to put their professional careers on the line, risking losing everything if the venture were to fail. These professionals formed the nucleus of a new Loma Linda-based clinical faculty.[10]

In anticipation of the opening of the new hospital, the Loma Linda University board of trustees made a request. They voted to urge the County of San Bernardino to complete the Anderson Street overpass at the Southern Pacific Railroad tracks by mid-1967. (That task was completed in mid-1968, only a year late.)[11] By that time passing trains had been stopping traffic in the area for more than 90 years.[12]

As the institution moved forward with the consolidation efforts, Reynolds justified the decision to move to Loma Linda. The move harmonized with the modern consensus that medical education could best be accomplished when (1) basic and clinical medical scientists work together in teaching and research in the battle against disease; and (2) the medical school is an integral part of a university, its faculty members a part of a larger multidiscipline teaching staff, and its students a part of a multi-interest academic community.[13]

While acknowledging times of conflict and turmoil through the years of consolidation, Hinshaw declared that his greatest strength lay in his belief that the School of Medicine was an institution with a sacred purpose: "I believed the Medical School was an institution of destiny in two ways: within the Church specifically, and in a large sense within Christianity. The Christian orientation in medical schools has essentially departed from us in this world. Most of them all have gone. We're it, and we were it during most of this period. What was left of a few of them evaporated along the trail and there is such a tight link in my mind between fundamental Christianity and fundamental Christian responsibility . . . that relates to healthcare and care of the sick, in a broad context."[14]

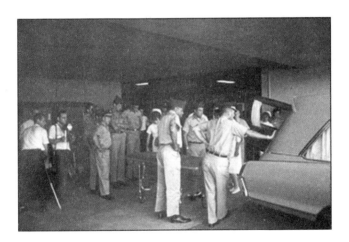

## Move-in Day

On July 9, 1967, in a disaster practice, 40 medics from the General Patton U.S. Army Reserve Center in Maywood, California, with buses and ambulances from the United States military, moved 125 patients from the hospital on the hill into the new facility, named "Loma Linda University Hospital." The move took three and a half hours, thirty minutes less than expected.[15]

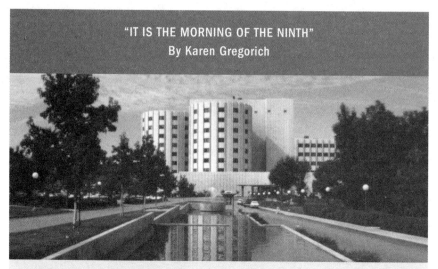

**"IT IS THE MORNING OF THE NINTH"**
By Karen Gregorich

**IT IS THE MORNING OF THE NINTH of July [1967].** Still thick with sleep, I struggle to open my eyes. There is someone in the room with me. The doctor is here already, before breakfast or morning temps, alert and smiling. I ask the time. It is ten of seven. The tone of his reply betrays some of the excitement he must be experiencing this proud day.

**NURSES ARE IN AND OUT CONSTANTLY.** I am fed, and my tray is hurriedly removed. I am tagged with an identifying band, labels are put on my suitcase and other belongings. Several nurses come to be sure my laboratory specimens are being handled correctly. Would I like to have a shower now? Can I hurry? No, there won't be time right now. I lie back in bed to rest after packing my belongings.

**A NURSE COMES WITH A WHEELCHAIR.** Her pace is brisk, her voice breathless. The time is now. I climb aboard and wheel rapidly down the hall, clutching my purse with one hand and with the other firmly gripping the wheelchair arm.

**AT THE ELEVATOR WE ENCOUNTER OUR FIRST HANG-UP.** We meet another patient, being moved in a bed, complete with oxygen tank. How will we manage the trip? Shall I climb out of the wheelchair and stand up? Shall they send me along with a wheelchair and oxygen tank, and let the bed and its occupant come later? The matter is pondered while we await the arrival of the elevator. The doors open to reveal another wheelchair patient, and the problem is solved: I will ride down first. In the basement, our little party meets more kindred spirits. There are several more wheelchair patients with their nurses, and others seated on the couch nearby. Someone says my wheelchair is needed, and I am helped onto the couch.

**WOMEN CLUTCHING LISTS AND PENCILS** run back and forth, asking questions of some and giving directions to others. Uniformed army men begin filing out of a nearby room, dropping paper cups and napkins into a trash receptacle at the door. Several of them group just beyond the doorway for directions from a campus police officer. Phrases float back to us: "Barton Road," "loading dock," "right turn." A young man and his pregnant wife enter hurriedly. The girl, obviously in pain, presses her hand first to her back, then her hip. She bends slightly forward. Her husband bangs impatiently on the elevator button for several minutes. Just as he looks around for someone to help, the elevator door opens. They step inside and are closed away.

**OUR GROUP IS MOVED OUTSIDE.** We huddle together about halfway between the building and the bus that we are to board. We are grateful for the shade while we wait. A doctor strolls toward us. Well, what are we waiting for, he wants to know. A nurse gives him a mock salute. The United States Army, sir! The young father-to-be hurries past us, clutching admission forms, presumably on the way to move his car. We continue to wait.

**WE ARE BOARDING THE ARMY-GREEN BUS.** I watch the procession as it enters. Men, women, of all ages and sizes, dressed in white terry robes, bright cotton wrappers, fussy negligees, loud pajamas; nurses in uniform, clutching suitcases, charts, medications, miscellaneous brown paper sacks, radios, even a plant or two.

**"WHERE DO YOU WANT ME TO SIT?"** "Pay your money and take your pick." "Sorry, I don't have a ticket!"

**A NURSE IS MOVING UP AND DOWN THE AISLE,** checking names and room numbers. But for the unusual garb and traveling gear, we appear to be a group of pleasure-bound tourists, most grinning broadly with expectation. Outside the bus, a doctor in a white coat is taking pictures.

**THE BIG BUS GROANS AND PUFFS.** We are under way at last. With some difficulty our driver navigates the steep, narrow road. I stifle a gasp as I glance out the window and look over the edge of the hill. We pass a sign which warns, "Do not enter. Severe tire damage." But the sharp prongs are down in anticipation of our passage, and we drive safely through.

**THE STREETS ARE LINED WITH CURIOUS SPECTATORS.** Several elderly ladies have set up a beach umbrella to protect them as they watch the proceedings. We press on. The giant, tan-colored building looms ahead. The driver backs into the emergency entrance and grinds the bus to a stop. There is a sense of confusion as the mass exodus begins. Courtesy is not apparent as the patients press toward the door. I sit quietly and wait until the bus is cleared. My nurse and I do not wait for a wheelchair, but make our way to the door of the building.

**A RIOT OF COLOR,** albeit somewhat subdued, greets us in the olive and gold stripes of the carpet. Slightly dazed by the effect, I follow my leader to the elevator. Another crush of wheelchairs, luggage, and bodies.

**THE ELEVATOR DOES NOT WISH TO COOPERATE.** It takes us down first, instead of up, and insists upon stopping at each floor and opening its doors for preliminary inspection. On the lobby level it reveals a panorama of rich, dark walnut.

**FOURTH FLOOR AT LAST.** Long corridors of windowless rooms. Unit 4200. More blends of soft color—golds, greens, browns, ivories. The rooms circle the nursing-station like the spokes of a wheel. A few patients are already here. My room is large, bright, tastefully decorated. The nurse opens the curtains. I'm instructed in the use of the various modern conveniences—the radio, the lights, the call button. Ice water is bought for me. I am settled.

**MY PART IN THE MOVE IS OVER,** and it has become just like any other hospital day, but I am filled with a sense of having taken part in something historic and significant.[16]

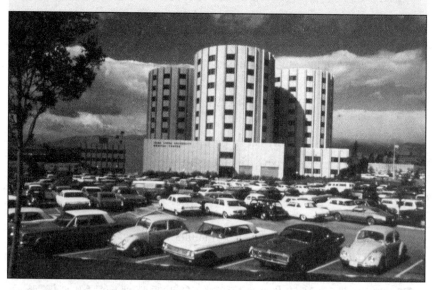

This view of Loma Linda University Medical Center from the south, before construction of Loma Linda University Children's Hospital and proton treatment center, clearly shows the towers built in a cloverleaf formation.

[1] "Design for the Future," *Loma Linda University Magazine*, July 1963, pp. 20-22.

[2] "1967: Goal for Completing University Medical Center," *University Scope*, January 31, 1964, p. 1.

[3] "Planners Complete Foundation Drawings for Medical Center," *University Scope*, May 1, 1964, p. 2; "Building Program Starts," *University Scope*, June 5, 1964, pp. 5, 12.

[4] "LLU Medical Center Ready for Start," *University Scope*, May 29, 1964, p. 1; June 19, 1964, pp. 1, 2.

[5] LLU board of trustees, minutes, September 27, 1966, p. 2. The $22.7-million structure was situated in what had been an orange grove along Barton Road.

[6] Tour notes compiled by Richard A. Schaefer, July 1966; "Plan New Medical Center Topping-Out January 25," *University Scope*, January 14, 1966, p. 1.

[7] Havstad had built Burden Hall, Evans Hall, Shryock Hall, the White Memorial Hospital, Risley Hall, the Library and Administration Building, the Clinical Laboratory/Pathology addition to the Loma Linda Sanitarium and Hospital, the School of Dentistry, Griggs Hall, the Student Activities Center (including the Campus Cafeteria), the Loma Linda Market, Kate Lindsay Hall, and Mortensen Hall. He also had built the Campus Hill Church and the White Memorial Church.

[8] Larry C. Havstad, oral history, January 25, 1971; Richard A. Schaefer, oral histories with Jimmy Havstad and Bud Heitschmidt, sons of Larry C. Havstad and Earl T. Heitschmidt, respectively, August 3, 2004.

[9] LLU board of trustees, minutes, May 25, 1965, p. 12; "Trustees Decide to Expand University Medical Center," *University Scope*, June 4, 1965, p. 1.

[10] Richard A. Schaefer, oral histories of David B. Hinshaw, M.D., November 2000, and Ellsworth E. Wareham, M.D., November 2002.

[11] Photo caption, *University Scope*, July 10, 1968, p. 8.

[12] LLU board of trustees, minutes, September 23, 1965, p. 6; John R. Signos, "The Yuma Main, Construction and Early Operation," *Beaumont Hill*, pp. 12, 13.

[13] Keld J. Reynolds, Ph.D., "The Academic Future of Loma Linda University," *Loma Linda University Magazine*, March 1964, p. 9.

[14] Merlin D. Burt and Petre Cimpoeru, oral history with David B. Hinshaw, Sr., M.D., July 16, 1996.

[15] "Rapid Transfer of 125 Patients Puts New Hospital in Operation," *University Scope*, July 12, 1967, p. 1.

[16] Karen Gregorich, "It Is the Morning of the Ninth," *Loma Linda University Magazine*, vol. 54, fall 1967, pp. 5-11.

# e shaped a healing ministry that has spread around the world!

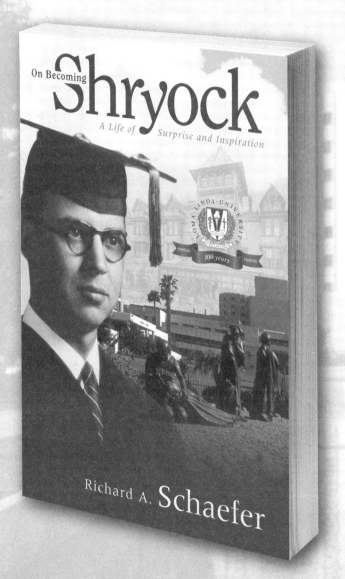

On Becoming **Shryock**
*A Life of* Surprise and Inspiration

LOMA·LINDA·UNIVERSITY
1905/06 · 100 years · 2005/06

Richard A. **Schaefer**

Richard A. Schaefer tells the story of Harold Shryock—master teacher, college administrator, trusted counselor, and prolific author—whose life spanned nearly a century and influenced a world. 978-0-8280-1889-0

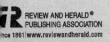
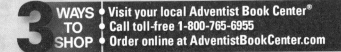

# Ellen White Series

by George R. Knight

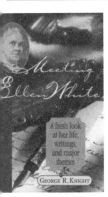
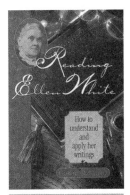
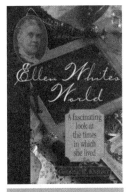
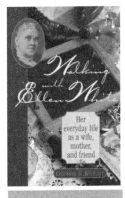

## Meeting Ellen White

ntroduces readers to e fascinating life and role of Ellen White. The author presents a iographical overview f her life and explores e major themes and tegories of her works. Especially helpful for new Adventists. Paperback. 978-0-8280-1089-4

## Reading Ellen White

A look at issues that have long been at the heart of Adventist understandings and misunderstandings of their prophet: the need for interpretive principles, her relation to the Bible, the purpose of her writings, and principles for interpreting and applying them. Paperback. 978-0-8280-1263-8

## Ellen White's World

This fascinating look at the world in which Ellen White lived provides a deeper appreciation and understanding of her writings. Includes many photographs and drawings illustrating life in the late 1800s and early 1900s. Paperback. 978-0-8280-1356-7

## Walking With Ellen White

Here is an intimate glimpse into Ellen White's personal life— her joys and struggles as a wife, mother, friend, and Christian. Paperback. 978-0-8280-1429-8 Also available in Spanish. 978-1-5755-4472-4

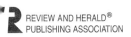

# Books That Feed Your Mind, Heart, and Soul

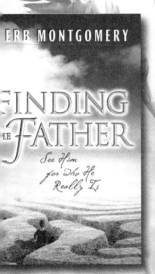

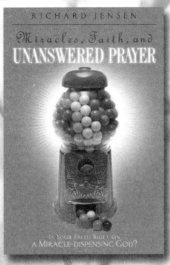

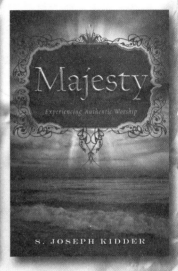

## ding the Father

rb Montgomery
pels Satan's lies that
w the character of
d and cause us to
rn the only one who
ly loves us. Encounter
d on an intensely
sonal level and
perience His life-
nging love. You'll
er see God the same
y again! 978-0-8280-
59-3

## Miracles, Faith, and Unanswered Prayers

Why does God answer
some prayers and not
others? Why do some
people seem to
experience miracles,
while others don't?
Does God play favorites?
Richard Jensen tackles
some of life's thorny
questions in this straightforward exploration of
Christian faith. 978-0-
8280-2015-2

## Majesty

Worship is a vibrant,
ongoing, authentic
encounter with God—a
life-changing experience!
Joseph Kidder shares
scriptural principles to
guide you into a genuine
worship experience that
will transform your soul
and leave you hungry for
God's presence. 978-0-
8280-2423-5